ALL YOU EVER WANTED TO KNOW

INDIAN DIETS

IN KIDNEY DISEASES

DR. SUNEETI ASHWINIKUMAR KHANDEKAR
DR. RACHANA JASANI

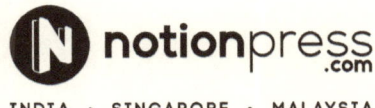

INDIA • SINGAPORE • MALAYSIA

Notion Press

Old No. 38, New No. 6
McNichols Road, Chetpet
Chennai - 600 031

First Published by Notion Press 2019
Copyright © Dr. Suneeti Ashwinikumar Khandekar 2019
All Rights Reserved.

ISBN 978-1-64760-672-5

This book has been published with all efforts taken to make the material error-free after the consent of the authors. However, the authors and the publisher do not assume and hereby disclaim any liability to any party for any loss, damage, or disruption caused by errors or omissions, whether such errors or omissions result from negligence, accident, or any other cause.

While every effort has been made to avoid any mistake or omission, this publication is being sold on the condition and understanding that neither the authors nor the publishers or printers would be liable in any manner to any person by reason of any mistake or omission in this publication or for any action taken or omitted to be taken or advice rendered or accepted on the basis of this work. For any defect in printing or binding the publishers will be liable only to replace the defective copy by another copy of this work then available.

Contents

Kidney Ki Baat *5*
About the Author 1 .... *7*
Message for Readers *9*
About the Author 2 .... *11*
Message for Readers *13*
Foreword *15*

Chapter 1	Introduction	17
Chapter 2	We are Different	20
Chapter 3	About Chronic Kidney Disease (CKD) and Nutrition	26
Chapter 4	Diet in CKD Stages 1 to 4	30
Chapter 5	Nutrition	33
Chapter 6	Home Food, Best Food	36
Chapter 7	All about Water	38
Chapter 8	Salt and Sodium	45
Chapter 9	All about Potassium	57

Contents

Chapter 10	Phosphorus Care	67
Chapter 11	Proteins	70
Chapter 12	Carbohydrates	81
Chapter 13	Fats	86
Chapter 14	Fruits	92
Chapter 15	Vegetables	95
Chapter 16	Food Items to Strictly Avoid – The Big No-No's	104
Chapter 17	Kidney Disease Diets – Myths and Facts	110
Chapter 18	Diet in Hemodialysis Patients	119
Chapter 19	Diet in Peritoneal Dialysis Patients	130
Chapter 20	Diabetes and Diet	136
Chapter 21	Diet in Kidney Stones	147
Chapter 22	Diet After Kidney Transplant	152
Chapter 23	Diet in Nephrotic Syndrome – The Protein Losing Kidney Problem	157
Chapter 24	Use of Ketoanalogues in Chronic Kidney Disease	160
Chapter 25	Kidney Friendly Recipes	164

(Chapters 18, 19, 21, 22, 23, 24 and 25 - Authored by Dr. Rachana Jasani)

Kidney *Ki Baat*

The seed of thought about writing a book on diet for kidney patients was sown way back in 2009, since I started practicing as a Nutritionist in Nagpur, Central India. There was general lack of awareness about the disease itself, leave apart the diet required in the disease.

And then to hear the prevailing myths surrounding the kidneys was a nightmare. I was a witness to several patients who succumbed to this illness due to malnutrition, stubbornly believing that proteins have to be completely avoided if one had kidney disease. To me, it showed the utter lack of knowledge about diet in kidney diseases.

I have counselled patients, conducted seminars with the help of Central India Nephrology Society, conducted seminars in schools, colleges and run awareness campaigns through print and digital media.

This book is dedicated to all those who have guided me, inspired and stood by me while writing.

Thank you Dr. Shobha Udipi. She instills thinking, a guide in true sense. Today, whatever I think, the way I think – are her ways of teaching and guiding. Thank you, madam, for everything.

Thank you Dr. Rachana Jasani for your long-term partnership, right from our college days, from the classrooms, labs, canteen, Hinduja hospital internship to writing this book.

Thank you Palash and Dr. Ashwinikumar Khandekar without whom, the seed of thought would have desiccated in the barren lands of hectic work schedules.

To all my patients- friends, who will surely know after reading this book, that this is everything that I counsel every patient when they meet me for the first time. Hours of counseling has helped me pen my words.

This book is for all those who met me and for all those, whom I wish to help fight CKD, to help them lead a quality life.

Thank You!

Warm Regards!

– Dr. Suneeti Ashwinikumar Khandekar

About the Author 1

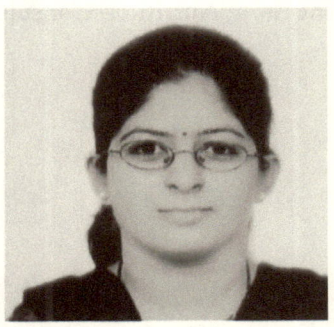

Dr. Suneeti Ashwinikumar Khandekar

Dr. Suneeti Ashwinikumar Khandekar MBBS, PGD in Dietetics and Clinical Nutrition (SNDT, Mumbai), MBA (Hospital Administration). After medical graduation and working in various esteemed hospitals and institutes, she studied in SNDT Mumbai, under the guidance of Dr. Shobha Udipi, Director, Post Graduate Studies and Research, SNDT, Juhu who was the president of the Indian Dietetic Association (IDA).

Her teaching experience include being a Lecturer in Medical Physiology at SNDT, Mumbai for the same course that she studied as student, faculty of Nutrition at Central India Nephrology Society, Nagpur, Central India. She also taught Pregnancy Nutrition at *Garbhasanskaar* classes in Nagpur and conducted pediatric and school nutrition programs in various schools across Nagpur.

She has a professional experience from the esteemed Hinduja Hospital, Mumbai where she worked as a dietitian. She has undertaken community nutrition work in the Aarey Milk Colony, Mumbai in 2006.

Currently, she is a Nutrition Consultant at Nagpur, Maharashtra.

Message for Readers

Dear Friends,

This book is for all who feel the need for Renal Diet.

This book is for **patients and their caregivers**. We have tried our best to keep the data and scientific language simple, so that our patients and their care givers would make the best use of the book.

This book is for **Students of Nutrition and Dietetics, Nursing students and Nursing staff in Dialysis Units and Post Kidney Transplant -Care Staff.** The scientific description shall help the subject of Renal Nutrition easy and understandable.

This book is for **Dialysis Technicians.** They are the people who give firsthand information to the dialysis patients, even before they reach the nutritionist. This book shall help the technicians to acquire and impart knowledge about renal nutrition to benefit the patients.

Please remember, this book serves as a general guideline for Kidney Diets. However, as medicine prescription is different from patient to patient, so is the diet. This book does not replace the dietary counselling of a Renal Dietitian.

About the Author 2

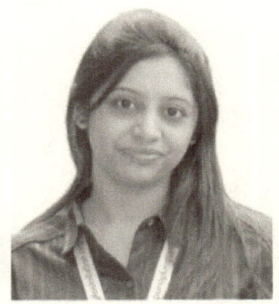

Dr. Rachana Jasani

Dr. Rachana Jasani, Ph.D, RD, has been trained at the esteemed institute Seth G S Medical College and KEM Hospital for dietary management of patients dealing with kidney diseases.

She has been practicing as a Consultant Renal Dietitian at Apex Kidney Care, a chain of dialysis centers across the country since 2008.

She has been an author for books named

"Nutrition Simplified for Dialysis patients" and

"Nutrition Simplified for transplant patients".

Message for Readers

"Dear Readers,

This book will help you gain an in-depth knowledge about what the role of diet is in kidney disease and how each aspect of nutrition can be managed. This book will also give you practical tips for making the necessary changes in your diet.

With this book, we aim to reach out to patients as well as caregivers struggling to find dietary advice.

However, this book contains only general dietary instructions, hence, it is important to understand that diet tips may vary from patient to patient as every individual is different. This book cannot replace the dietary counselling of a Renal Dietitian".

Foreword

In a hectic work schedule of a kidney doctor, patients expect that the doctor talks at length on the diet planning. However, the best that the doctor can do is to refer the patient to a kidney dietitian. Having known Dr. Suneeti as an avid counsellor, it was only natural to think that those counselling sessions should now take shape of a book that the patients can refer to repeatedly and the doctor can now hand over a copy saying, "this is my diet counselling to you!" Dr. Suneeti has found an accomplished partner in Dr. Rachana Jasani to complement her in completing the task.

Diet plays an important role in the management of most non communicable chronic diseases. In fact, the moment patient is diagnosed with a disease, the first question that is posed to the doctor is, "Was it because of something I ate?" And after a long narration by the doctor explaining that may be that was not the case, the subsequent question is, "Now, what should I not eat?"

These beliefs are deep rooted in our minds from an era prior to scientific advancements. In ancient times, if one developed a disease one would try to correlate it with what they ate the previous day and then try to avoid it in the future, thinking it might help. That's how the concept of

Foreword

parhez (abstinence from certain food items) came to stick. Patients feel the consultation with the doctor is incomplete until the doctor enumerates at least a couple of items of *parhez*!

With progress in medical science, we have now reached a stage where we can pinpoint to different constituents of food playing any role in non-communicable diseases like chronic kidney disease. We know we don't have to blindly leave out certain food items from our diet. It is now, more about planning to include food items rather than leave them out simply out of fear.

Diet management in kidney disease is an area where patients have a plethora of misbeliefs and misconceptions. Family doctors and general practitioners are not immune to these misconceptions and may unwittingly reinforce them. This book serves to address these misconceptions by explaining scientific concepts behind each aspect of diet planning in kidney diseases.

This book says it is possible to have a normal diet even if one is suffering from kidney disease. Moderation remains the key. Let the world of a kidney patient be not all about *parhez*!

– Dr. Ashwinikumar Khandekar

CARE Hospital, Nagpur

Chapter 1

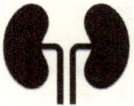

Introduction

"Doctor, my reports say that my kidneys are failing. What should I eat now?"

This is the usual beginning of our conversation.

The patients ask with an anxious look in their eyes.

They have a lot of questions. They are curious to know as to what more is in store for them.

This is common! Be it an elderly lady or a chemistry student, a young mother of a 6-year-old, a tall and handsome executive or gentleman with already pre-existing illnesses, someone with coronary bypass surgery or angioplasty.

All are similarly anxious when they meet me for the first time.

Kidney diseases have such an impact on our minds, that we all become cautious or extra-cautious about everything we do.

Diet is no exception. It is a priority nowadays. Patients of all age groups tend to find information on the internet, read books and seek advices.

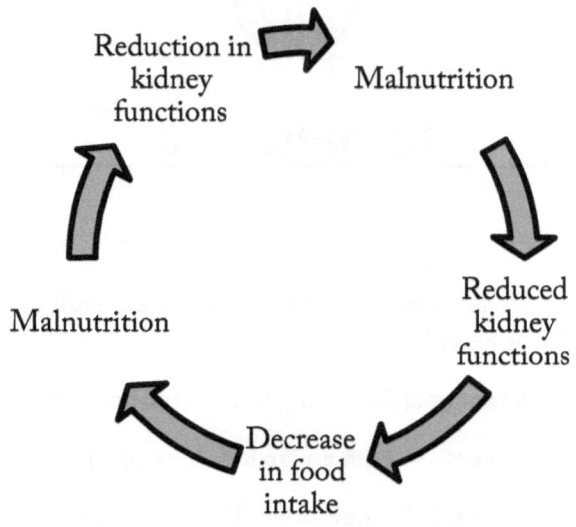

The Vicious cycle of Malnutrition and Reduction in Kidney Functions

In all such cases, expert and authentic advice needs to be sought in pursuit of preventing further damage to the kidneys or to delay the progression of kidney disease.

However, all that the majority of patients know is that we have to religiously follow some kind of a Kidney-friendly diet or the Renal diet.

Breaking News! Renal diet, per se, is not just boiled, no salt no taste food!

In fact, kidney disease diet or the 'Renal diet' is really a diet with plenty of options to choose from. Many tasty

Introduction

recipes can be made which we never thought was allowed with kidney disease.

It should always be kept in mind that every individual is different.

Every patient has different lifestyle, food habits, education status, economic status and most important – disease status.

The doctor prescribes medicines to all chronic kidney disease patients. These medicines are based on their parameters as height, weight, pulse, blood pressure, blood parameters and the stage of kidney failure by estimating Glomerular filtration Rate, the eGFR.

As every medical prescription is different, so is every dietary prescription or advice.

Remember, as medicines change or their doses change according to the kidney "status", so should the diet.

This book is a small attempt to reach patients with the general guidelines about Chronic Kidney Disease (CKD) diet.

Chapter 2

We are Different

We are Indians.

Salute!

Proud to be an Indian!

We are different.

We differ in everything.

This is in reference to the rest of the world.

India is culturally and cuisine-wise diverse.

Some parts of India are warm and humid. Some are hot and dry. At high altitudes, we experience extreme cold weathers! From Kashmir to Kanyakumari, we have differing weather conditions. And according to the weather conditions, we plan our daily diet.

Thus, monsoons are greeted with chai-pakoras, in winters we relish hot puris and summers are full of homemade cold drinks or lassi or buttermilk or raw mango drinks.

We cook variety and in variety of ways.

We all know we need to eat a

- Carbohydrate source, i.e. rice or wheat or *jowar* or maize or both,
- A protein source like *dals* or chicken or sprouts,
- Fat source such as oils and *ghee*,
- Milk and milk products as in *kheers*, curds, buttermilk, *paneer*,
- Minerals as in salts and spices,
- Vitamins and fiber in vegetables and fruits.
- Do not miss out on water as an integral part of our diets.

In an Indian meal, can we separate various ingredients of a recipe into one being a carbohydrate source and the other as a protein source?

No! We cannot!

We cook in a blending form which mixes everything together.

The combination thus cooked is our divine experience, Our Indian Food!

Every Indian household has a different recipe as a traditional, family inheritance.

For example, given raw rice

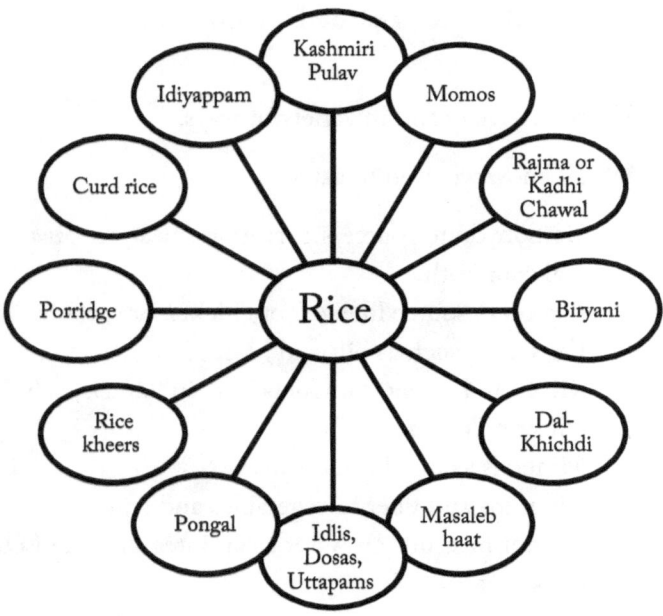

- A Kashmiri will make a saffron based *Kashmiri pulav*,
- *Momos* shall be made in the North east,
- A Punjabi will cook *Rajma chawal or Kadhi* chawal,
- A Lucknowi will cook a mouth-watering *biryani*,
- Gujaratis will make delicious *khichadi*,
- Maharashtrians will cook *plain dal bhaat* or spicy, vegetable-laden *masale-bhaat*,
- South Indians will make *idlis, dosas, uthappams*.
- Karnatakis will have curd rice or sweet rice,
- Tamilians will convert rice into *Idiyappam* (rice noodles),
- Keralites will make rice *kheers*.

And the list goes on.

We are Different

If just raw rice can be cooked in so many ways, then think about the wide range of food grains we eat!

Another peculiarity of Indian cooking is that Mrs. Veena's *sambar* may not taste like that of Mrs. Shrilaxmi and so is the case with the *parathas* at Pummy aunty's and *puran* polis at the Sahastrabuddhes.

The point is – we Indians are unique. We use the same ingredients in different ways. We come up with our best culinary skills. So, each household has a different taste to the same menu.

Hence, we should discuss our food habits in details with our Renal nutritionist. That will help us plan a proper kidney-friendly and a patient friendly diet.

Another important aspect of our culture is the festivals and fasts and the food items associated with it. These also should be taken into consideration.

Why festivals and fasts?

Well, fasting, without food and water – staying empty stomach the whole day – is not advisable at all to patients.

But when it comes to festivals and fasts given our traditional and religious backgrounds, the patients find it difficult to stay away and hence this aspect should also be included in diet planning (options and exceptions are always to be considered). We have grown up in this environment, are brought up in a culture where festivals and traditions are an integral part of our daily routine.

Most important aspect of this is to help the CKD patients to lead a quality and normal or near normal life. (**Quality of Life Index-QOLI**)

Caution – Do not fall into the trap of the common statements made by our near or dear ones," Have little, it won't harm you."

Statutory Warning: The statements and sentiments of force-feeding are dietetically dangerous.

Thomas Stearns Eliot, a famous English poet, in his poem "The Rock" quotes,

"Where is the life we have lost in living?

Where is the wisdom we have lost in knowledge?

Where is the knowledge we have lost in information?"

With all the technological advances and change, is mankind happier or wiser than it was 100 years ago?

We need to live!

We need to read and gain knowledge!

We need to apply that knowledge with wisdom in our lives practically!

Let's use knowledge to live a quality of life, which we otherwise would have lived anyways, quality or not!

Think not about the problem alone,

Think that this is a situation

I need to tackle, solve!

It's like the levels in a computer game. We are stuck inside till we successfully cross the level and reach the higher level. Difficulties increase as we complete levels and reach the top to be a winner!

In CKD cases, a winner is the one who leads a quality, healthy lifestyle despite knowing to be having the problem.

Be a Winner!

Let's get started with the basics of CKD nutrition.

Chapter 3

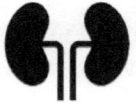

About Chronic Kidney Disease (CKD) and Nutrition

Chronic Kidney Disease (CKD) is a decline in the kidney's ability to remove waste products.

This is reflected by

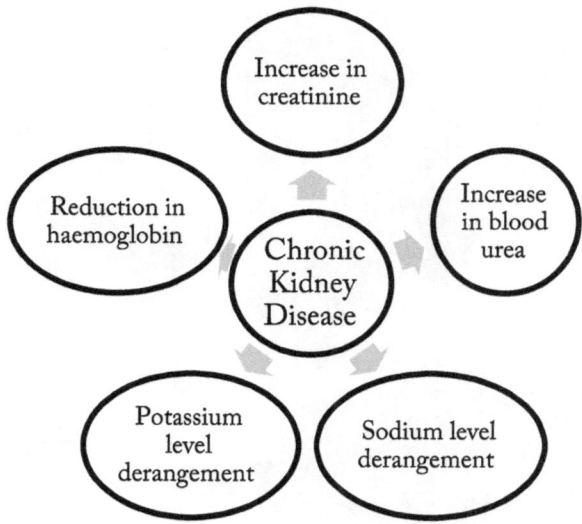

About Chronic Kidney Disease (CKD) and Nutrition

- An increase in serum creatinine level,
- Increase in blood urea level and
- Sometimes derangement in blood minerals as sodium, potassium and
- Reduction in Hemoglobin level (Anemia).

Purpose of Nutrition Care in CKD

1. To maintain Nutritional status.

- To have a well-balanced diet within the restrictions advised.
    a. Sometimes, the gut or emotions may tell otherwise, but stick to the diet plan.
    b. Sticking to the diet helps the patient, in the long run, to stay healthy.
- Taste? Major issue!
    a. The change in diet will bring restrictions in amounts of salt and spices, certain vegetables and recipes and of outside eating.
    b. Metabolic changes in CKD lead to taste changes or aversions.

Remember, taste is only limited to a small but important organ, tongue.

We should be brave to neglect its craving for taste.

Instead, we should eat the important nutrients, cooked in the way advised by our nutritionist and gulp it down like good boys and girls.

It is for us to stay healthy.

Once we gulp our food down the throat, the gut recognizes it as nutrients or chemicals. Not as *biryani* or gravy or plain bland *khichdi*.

All we need to do is eat nutrients to stay healthy or delay the progression of chronic kidney disease.

(Do not worry! We shall discuss some yummy, tasty, kidney friendly recipes later).

2. To slow the progression of renal failure and possibly delay the need for maintenance dialysis.

- By religiously following the food, water and medicine prescriptions by our doctor and nutritionist.
- Plan a proper exercise schedule, with the help of a certified trainer, to keep fit.

3. To prevent or minimize uremic symptoms by reducing the accumulation of nitrogenous waste products.

- By following protein consumption as per the advice.
- Eating the right quantity and right quality of protein helps minimize sense of nausea, vomiting and giddiness or lethargy.

4. To control hypertension by minimizing fluid and electrolyte disturbances.

- Fluid - intake needs to be measured.
- Fluids include plain water as well as other liquids taken all throughout the day in the form of tea, dals, vegetables, fruits and the water used in cooking.

About Chronic Kidney Disease (CKD) and Nutrition

- Salt and sodium restrictions by eating salt as advised, potassium and phosphorus restricted diet needs to be followed for taking a balanced diet.

Points to Remember

- ✓ **Nutritious and balanced diet to be consumed.**
- ✓ **Medicines, food, water intake and exercise should be performed under expert advice and guidance.**
- ✓ **Special attention to be given on protein intake.**
- ✓ **Keep a check on salt, potassium and phosphorus intake to prevent hypertension and electrolyte imbalances.**
- ✓ **Measure 24 hours salt and water intake.**

Chapter 4

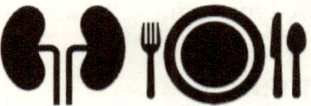

Diet in CKD Stages 1 to 4

We shall name this as the CKD diet.

The Stage 5 diet shall be named Dialysis (Hemodialysis and Peritoneal Dialysis) diet.

Recommended Dietary Education Should Take Place Over 3 Visits

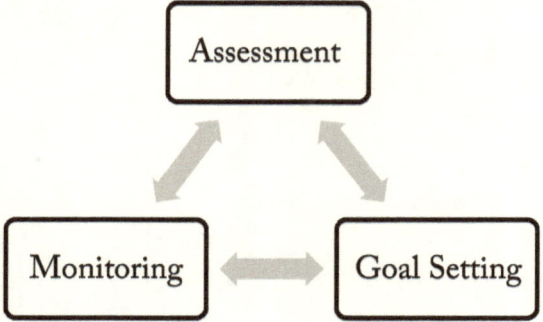

1. Assessment

- There should be a detailed discussion about the patient's condition
- History of illness

- Recent blood reports
- Detailed daily diet history
- Diet diary, a record keeping for 3 to 7 days
- Dietary likes and dislikes, religious beliefs and the societal implications.

2. Goal setting

After assessing the situation, dietary goals need to be set for:

- Calories
- Proteins
- Water intake
- Sodium (salt intake) and Potassium
- Phosphorus
- Carbohydrates, fats and fibre.

3. Monitoring

- Daily diet record keeping.
- Changes to be suggested every 15 days, taking into account the general condition and blood parameters of the patient.
- Once the diet is adjusted according to the blood parameters, the patients may continue on the same diet till their next nephrologist visit and/ or blood tests done.

This should be done steadily, with every detail discussed with the nutritionist.

It is a two-way process, and no one should be in haste, as we all know, Haste makes Waste.

Points to Remember

- ✓ Diet advice is an essential aspect in CKD.
- ✓ Assessment, goal setting and monitoring are the keys to a complete renal diet.
- ✓ Regular diet follow-up, once in three months, along with the recent blood parameter reports, is required.
- ✓ Medicines, diet and exercise are the key to quality of life in CKD.

Let us discuss the basics of CKD diet.

Chapter 5

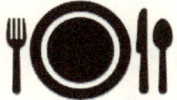

Nutrition

What is Nutrition?

Nutrition is the science of food and its interaction in us to promote and maintain good health.

Food is the necessity of living.

"Anna hey Poorna Brahma."

We need food to survive, grow and maintain health.

Sheilah Graham says

"Food is the most primitive form of comfort."

What are Nutrients?

(That we lose in cooking and overcooking.)

Nutrients supply nourishment.

They are required in right amounts.

They must be taken regularly.

There are six general classes of nutrients.

They are

- carbohydrates,
- proteins,
- fats,
- vitamins,
- minerals and
- water.

And an important element – Fiber- though not having any calories, but its presence is of utmost importance in smooth absorption and functioning of the nutrients.

Of these, some are essential nutrients without which an individual cannot function.

Each one of the nutrients and fiber are important for our body.

These nutrients, present in food, may be divided into macro nutrients and micro nutrients.

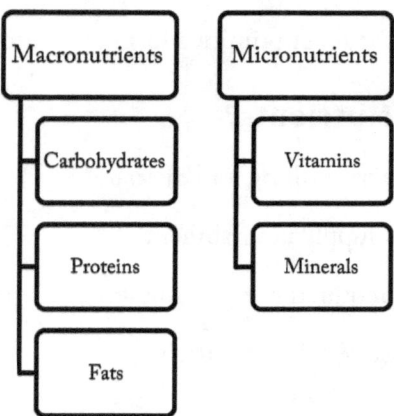

Macro Nutrients

- These are carbohydrates, proteins and fats.
- They are often called as 'proximate principles', because they form the main bulk of the food.

Micro Nutrients

- These are vitamins and minerals.
- They are called micronutrients because they are required in small amounts.

Points to Remember

- ✓ **Carbohydrates: Cereals, sugars, jaggery, potatoes and other root vegetables, fruits.**
- ✓ **Proteins: Milk and milk products, eggs, chicken, fish, dals and pulses.**
- ✓ **Fats: Oils, ghee, butter.**
- ✓ **Vitamins: Fruits and vegetables.**
- ✓ **Minerals: Fruits and vegetables.**
- ✓ **Water: Plain water and other liquids.**
- ✓ **Fibre: Whole grains, sprouts, fruits and vegetables.**

Chapter 6

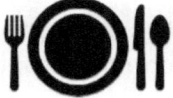

Home Food, Best Food

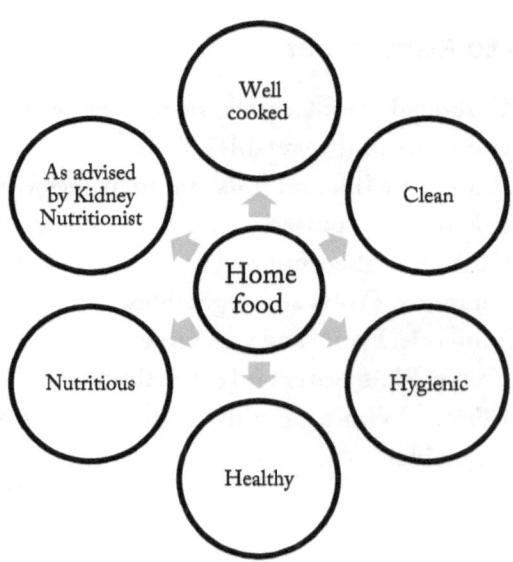

Home Food Benefits

Home food is:

- Well cooked
- Clean

Home Food, Best Food

- Hygienic
- Healthy
- Nutritious and
- According to all the methods of preparation advised by the renal nutritionist.

So, there should be no doubts, no second thoughts.

Home food should be in the mind and on the plate.

This principle should be followed not only by patients, but by the caretakers and caregivers who accompany patients.

Outside eating, occasionally, is acceptable.

The outside food we choose occasionally, should also be as well cooked, clean, hygienic, healthy and nutritious as home-cooked food.

Irony is we expect home food should be as tasty as hotel menu, while in the hotel menu, we try to search for homely preparations.

Still, Home Food - Best Food!

Points to Remember

- ✓ **Always eat home food. All nutrients are preserved.**
- ✓ **We know what goes in that *gravy*, soup or *chapati*.**
- ✓ **Maintain kitchen hygiene. Wash all utensils, gadgets, knives after every use.**
- ✓ **Quality of raw ingredients used can be controlled.**
- ✓ **Recipes are cooked according to the kidney diet guidelines.**

Chapter 7

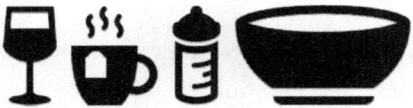

All about Water

Chronic Kidney Disease progresses with loss of kidney functions.

Decrease in urine output happens gradually.

If we happen to drink excess water at this stage, the water starts accumulating in our body.

Weight gain happens to the extent of 3 kg before any swelling is visible. Beyond this, swelling appears in the feet, ankles, legs.

Gradually the water accumulates in the abdominal cavity and lungs, leading to breathlessness.

Rise in blood pressure can also be a major consequence.

Thus, the symptoms are:

All about Water

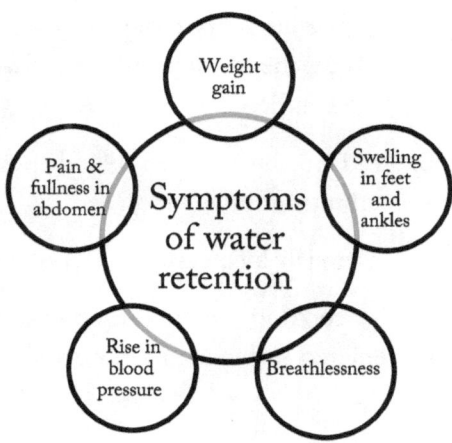

- Weight gain
- Swelling in the ankles and feet
- Breathlessness
- Rise in blood pressure
- Pain and fullness in the abdomen.

In such cases, water intake needs to be restricted.

Fluid intake is often mistaken as only water intake.

When the doctor says to drink 1.5 liters of fluids in a day, we drink that much of plain water without measuring the other 'fluids' that we are consuming - the tea, milk, buttermilk, curry in vegetables, not to forget the thin *dal*. Remember, water is used for cooking rice and *rotis* as well.

All this adds to a huge sum of water.

It is a common problem that patients have swelling on the feet and yet they continue drinking so much of fluids.

With reducing urine output day by day, the water retained in our body reaches to such an extent that the heart finds it too much to handle.

This may lead to increase in blood pressure and difficulties in breathing and much more.

Please act consciously by measuring all types of fluids.

Remember, for cooking, we require water and all these chemicals, once entered in the stomach start showing their "properties".

Let us discuss about Water intake.

Boiled or Filtered Water

Boiling water is water that boils till 'rolling boil' for 20 minutes in a wide-mouthed container. This is done to remove germs from water, for disease prevention.

By the term **filtered water**, we mean the water obtained by standard purification methods with Reverse Osmosis (RO) filter, charcoal filter and lead filter.

These filters should be properly maintained, and their servicing should be done regularly and religiously.

The old-style candle filters should no longer be relied upon.

Common questions asked are:

All about Water

- How much water?
- How to measure water?

We need to know the exact amount of fluids that we are consuming in one day, that is in 24 hours.

If our nephrologist has asked us to take, for example, 1.5 liters of fluids in a day, it should include everything that is liquid in nature,

- Tea
- Milk
- *Dal*
- Buttermilk
- Plain water that we drink and
- Even the water required for cooking.

So, how do we go about our daily fluid intake in the above example ?

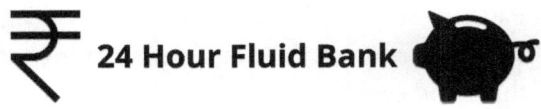

24 Hour Fluid Bank

- To begin with –
    - Fill water in a one-litre bottle full and
      Another one-litre bottle half or get a half litre bottle.

This becomes our "24-hour Fluid Bank" or "Daily Fluid Allowance".

To utilize this fluid bank

- Now, to make tea, for example, use water from this bottle so that we know the remaining amount of water
- Or, discard the amount of water equal to the amount of tea we drank, from our daily fluid quota,
- We should implement the above method without fail, each time we have something liquid.

To make this fluid bank last 24 hrs

- Use **smaller glasses** for drinking.
- Schedule the **medicines with major meals** as far as possible, so that we save on additional water intake to take our medicines.

- To **control or manage thirst**,

  - Engage in activities, which helps us to forget our problems (thirst, in this case) and keeps us occupied and happy.
  - Patients with **diabetes** should keep their **blood sugars in control**. Rise in sugars also increases the thirst and eventually water intake.

For winters and cool weather, this plan works.

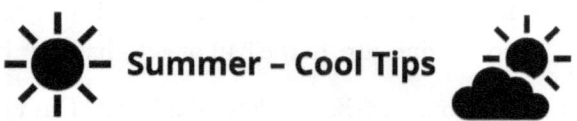 **Summer – Cool Tips**

Indian summers and early monsoons are hot and humid.

We follow these rules of measurement of water:

All about Water

- Additional water intake should be avoided as far as possible.
- Stay indoors in summers, stay in coolers, fans, air-conditioners.
- When thirsty, you may
    - Just gargle and spit out water or
    - Wet your lips.
    - Use wet towels.
- Some crystal sugars or " *Cham-chami shakkar*" can be kept in the mouth so that you salivate, and it quenches thirst. (Not for patients with Diabetes)
- Mouth fresheners, cardamom (*Eliachi*), one clove (*Laung*) piece or some dried ginger (*sunth*) can be placed in the mouth, to prevent dryness of mouth. Remember to change the ingredient kept in the mouth after every 3–4 hours. Also, it should be avoided during night-times or while taking naps during daytime, so that we do not unknowingly choke. Also, the insides of the mouth – the oral cavity lining called the mucosa – may get irritated and injured by constantly keeping something in the mouth.
- Fruit-Ice: Fruits which are allowed for CKD (Guava, Apple, Pear, Papaya, Pineapple- quantity as discussed with your renal nutritionist) can be cut into small pieces, put in the freezer compartment of your refrigerators and when frozen, can be enjoyed as ice-candy to quench thirst.
- Eat less salty foods, avoid extra salt in salads, rice, *rotis, puris* or *parathas*.

- Avoid pickles, *papads, chutneys, sherbets* which are rich in salts, sugars, preservatives and water. These food preservatives increase our thirst.
- Eat foods which are low in spices, oils and ghee. Avoid oily, spicy and fried items.
- Eat foods which are high in fibre, fresh, as raw as possible, not overcooked.

These summer tips may help prevent the large water intakes and thus help us in many ways.

Points to Remember

- ✓ **Make a 24-hour fluid bank.**
- ✓ **Fill in one litre bottle. Use water from this bottle/bank.**
- ✓ **Follow the "Half glass initiative."**
- ✓ **Schedule medicines with breakfast, lunch or dinners to avoid extra water intake.**
- ✓ **Strictly control blood sugars to prevent thirst.**
- ✓ **During summers, stay indoors.**
- ✓ **Gargle with water when thirsty.**
- ✓ **Use sugars crystals (not in case of diabetes), fruit ice or mouth fresheners.**
- ✓ **Limit salt intake to prevent thirst.**
- ✓ **Avoid oily, fatty and spicy meals.**

Chapter 8

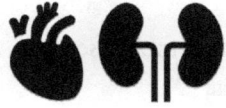

Salt and Sodium

Sodium in our blood

- Helps retain water in our body
- Helps maintain blood-pressure.

The levels of sodium in the blood are maintained by our kidneys.

Failing kidneys, as in Chronic Kidney Disease, leads to sodium retention in our body.

Normal Serum Sodium Range – 135–145 meq/l

Sodium, when exceeds in our blood, is the the main reason for water retention in our body.

- How does Sodium act?
- What is the relation of Salt intake and water retention?

Before answering these questions, let us understand something about thirst mechanism of our body.

Thirst Mechanism

"Salt" chemically means sodium chloride.

When we eat salty foods, sodium is released in blood after the food is digested.

This sodium-rich, circulating blood goes to the brain.

In our brain, there are sensors which sense this rise in blood sodium levels.

These sensors send signals to the other part of our brain.

'Knock-knock, sodium levels high.'

This other part is the "thirst-center".

The thirst-center gets activated.

It sends signals to our throat.

Brain asks for water intake.

In simple words, 'our throat feels dry and we feel thirsty'.

And we rush towards plain water.

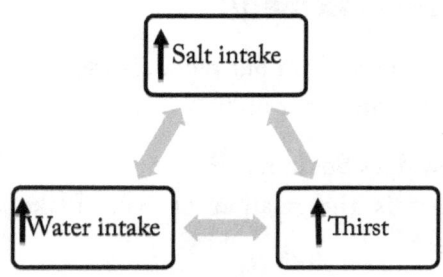

The Vicious Salt-Thirst-Water intake cycle

So, more the Salt intake, more the thirst, more the water intake.

We quench our thirst till the point where there is normalization of blood sodium levels. Thirst mechanism makes us drink water slightly in excess of needs of our body. This is because we cannot 'produce' water inside our body. We have to rely on intake from outside. The balance is quickly and consistently achieved by the normal kidneys by 'throwing out' the excess water.

With failing kidneys, thirst mechanism is intact, but the route to throw out excess water is 'blocked'. This leads to the edema (swelling in feet, ankles, legs, hands, puffiness of face, shortness of breath due to water being collected in the open air spaces in our lungs), rise in blood pressures and the related problems.

Hence, the advice to patients with CKD is to reduce salt intake.

Less salt, less thirst sensation, less water intake or say optimum water intake, no edema or at least lesser chances of getting edema.

Salt Restriction in Food

There comes a list with a warning to stay away…

Salty foods …. Stay away….

Stay away from

- *Papads*

- *Seviyas*
- Pickles
- *Chutneys*
- *Chaat* masalas
- Ready to eat items like salted popcorn, *sev, chiwda, chakli,* chips, wafers
- Bakery items and biscuits which have baking soda
- Salted nuts, salted butter, cheese
- Sauces, ketchups, jams, jellies, instant noodles, macaroni etc.
- Salted dried fishes and red meat
- Dried vegetables
- Green leafy vegetables with high sodium content as spinach, fenugreek, radish, beet
- Antacids and laxatives.

Salt is the best preservative.

It makes food stay fresh and eatable for long times.

Stay away from these food items to reduce salt intake.

Eat fresh, stay healthy!

Hidden Sodium

We all learnt it in school,

"All that glitters is not Gold".

On similar lines,

"All Sodium is not Salty."

By this, I mean the sodium rich chemicals used as preservatives in many of our favorite eatables.

They may not taste salty, or may not have any taste, but they are sodium-based.

The List:

1. Baking powder and soda. (Sodium Bicarbonate)
2. Sauces and ketchups. (Sodium Benzoate)
3. Jellies, desserts, beverages. (Sodium Citrate)
4. Ice-creams and chocolate milk. (Sodium Alginate)
5. Dry fruits color and coatings. (Sodium Sulphite)
6. Artificial sweeteners. (Sodium Saccharide)
7. Meat preservatives. (Sodium Nitrate)

As discussed earlier, this sodium, when enters our gut, shows its real properties.

There is rise in blood sodium levels, then follows the thirst and drinking of water and hence, the water retention.

So, we need to stay away from these too.

Now arises the frequently asked questions:

- Which salt to eat?
- How much salt to eat?
- How do we know how much salt we are eating?
- "We do not use salt in salads, nor do we use salt-shakers, we eat less salt." Is the argument usually.

Let us learn this step by step...

- **Which salt to eat?**
  - "*Shudh*, free flow, refined, iodized, *safed namak*".
    - ✓ No, I am not endorsing any salt brand here.
    - ✓ It's just what I want to stress on.
    - ✓ **Salt means 'Sodium Chloride'.**
    - ✓ All these properties are there in all the branded, refined, iodised salts, sea salts.
    - ✓ Please use Common Salt, the white one, packaged and branded.
    - ✓ We simply need to consume the chemical "Sodium Chloride".
  - Salt Substitutes:
    - ✓ What if we use other types of salts? Another query.
    - ✓ This discussion now includes rock salt, black salt, salts used during fasts, *sanchal* or *sanchar namak*- the non-refined salts, the "*desi*" way or
    - ✓ Low Sodium salts, Light salts and others, the "medical" way.

Dear friends, remember the line we read a few minutes ago, "All Sodium is not Salty".

On similar lines, "All Salty is not Sodium".

Stumped!!!

These are known as '**Salt Substitutes**' in medical language.

Sodium – when replaced by other chemical as Potassium – becomes Potassium Chloride, with Magnesium becomes Magnesium Chloride, with Calcium becomes Calcium Chloride.

All these taste more or less like common salt, the white, sea-salt that we consume.

In CKD we need to eat less sodium to prevent water retention in the body.

Similarly, other chemical salts too get retained in the body due to the failing filtration processes in the kidneys.

Potassium salts lead to increase in the levels of blood potassium.

That can prove dangerous, I repeat 'dangerous' for the heart as it can can cause arrhythmias.

An Arrhythmia is an abnormal heart rhythm.

Arrhythmias can produce a broad range of symptoms, from barely perceptible to cardiovascular collapse.

So, for want of salt, a heart turned at fault.

Save! Save!

Cut to Take 1... Action... *Shudh*, free flow, refined, iodized, common salt should be eaten.

How Much Salt to Eat?

But we put less salt while cooking!

Usual argument, very much routine.

Do we measure salt as in grams?

No! not even as in 'teaspoons.'

We just use fingers and hands on to that salt container, dig salt with our fingertips and pour, literally pour, till our taste buds are filled with the salty flavor.

Now that the rule is to reduce salt for the good here, we should follow certain practices, which means to stop certain culinary routines as:

No adding salt in:

- Dough,
- *Parathas* of all kinds,
- *Bhakri, puri, naan, bhatura,* rice.

But then, what would it taste like?

Simple logic dear friends!

We do not eat them as alone. We eat all these carbs with *dals*, vegetables, *raitas*. All these supplies are with salt.

So, stop adding salt to the carbohydrate bases.

- No adding salt to salads. Eat them fresh, relish their original tastes.
- Some add salt to cut fruits too! Stop!

How do we measure the salt allowance for the whole day?

- A pinch made of Thumb, Index and Middle finger measurement of the above description common salt is close to "one gram". Remember, outer sides of the *chutki* or pinch need to be wiped off.

Salt and Sodium

- So, a CKD stage 1–4 patient can eat common salt as advised by the Nephrologist, measuring it with his/her own fingers. Six to eight grams of salt means 6–8 pinches of salt per day or as advised.
- Keep this measured salt ready every morning.

Now, let us have a look at the routine cooking techniques.

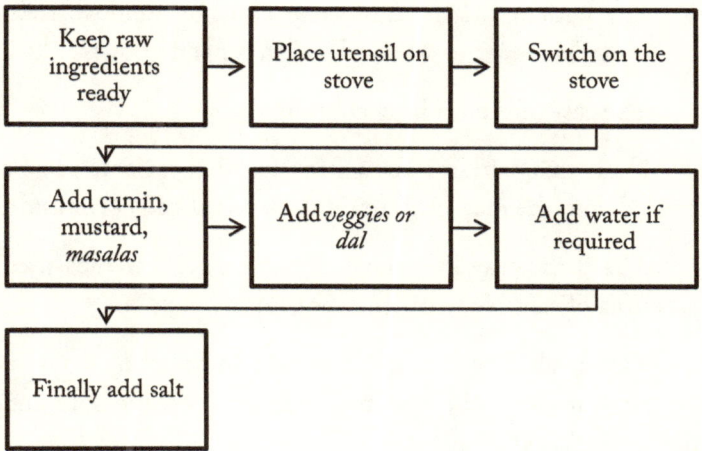

Basic Cooking Technique

We all know that at first the raw material is kept ready, then we switch on the stove, pour oil in utensil, then the cumin, mustard seeds and *masalas*, then vegetables or *dal*, add water if required, then cook. No salt yet, right?

Finally, when done or almost done, the last to come in is salt and sugar to taste. But wait before we do so.

Here is the **breakpoint** in this cooking session.

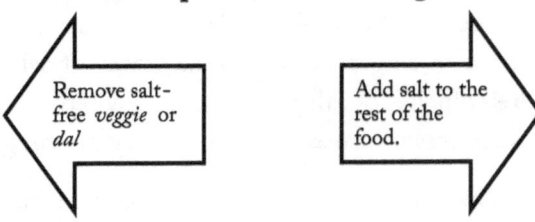

For the patient in the family, we can now remove their portion of salt-free *veggies* and *dals* in separate bowls.

The rest of the cooking continues.

Now, this salt-free food kept for the patient, can be treated with the measured amounts of salt already kept aside.

That's the way it is done. Exact way to eat measured amounts of salt. Not a pinch more, not a pinch less.

These salt-free preparations help in so many ways to protect our weak kidneys from rise in blood pressure and rise in workload on heart.

- As far as taste is concerned, everything goes in our tummies and becomes chemicals, some useful and some harmful.
- Nah, I cannot be too cruel here!

Let us explore some 'allowed' items for taste enhancements.

Try and use these taste enhancers in place of salt in foods and discover a unique taste. I am sure, you won't miss salt.

- *Amchoor* (dried green mango powder).
- *Pudina* (mint), dried or fresh, amounts - very little.

Salt and Sodium

- *Dhaniya* or *dhaniya* powder (coriander).
- *Jeera* (cumin seeds).
- Ginger.
- Garlic.
- Celery.
- White vinegar (only a few drops).
- For any preparation that has a sour taste of its own, we can minimize the salt to be added.

Remember, according to the nephrologists, the formula for calculating Salt and Water intake used by them is,

For first 500 ml of water that you drink, salt intake allowed is One gram.

For every next 250 ml of water, one gram of salt is allowed.

Thus,

500 ml = 1 gm

250 ml = 1 gm

250 ml = 1 gm.

So, if the fluid allowed is 1000 ml or 1 litre, salt allowance is 3 gram per day.

Strict are the rules, strict is the calculation.

But this is all to prevent water retention and edema and prevent the dangers of water excess in the body.

Water is Life, please do not make it Life-Threatening.

Remember, salt is very essential for maintaining blood pressure and eventually, the balance of our body.

So, completely avoiding salt intake may also prove dangerous.

Enjoy the unique flavor of each ingredient in the recipes, rather than unnecessarily stuffing it with spices and salt.

Greats like Vinoba Bhave and Baba Amte have described this unique, original form of cuisine as Satvik Aahaar.

"Satvik Aahaar, Ucch Vichaar."

Points to Remember

- ✓ **Use Sodium chloride salt (common salt, white sea salt).**
- ✓ **Avoid salt substitutes.**
- ✓ **Avoid salty, ready to eat foods and foods with preservatives.**
- ✓ **More the salt, more the thirst, more the water intake and more the swelling. Avoid extra salt.**
- ✓ **A pinch made of index, middle finger and thumb holds approximately one gram of free flow, refined salt.**
- ✓ **Measure salt.**

Chapter 9

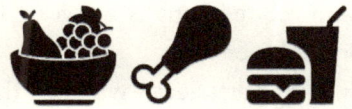

All about Potassium

Potassium is a mineral present in every living cell. It is chemically known as Kalium, hence the symbol "K" for potassium.

The Vital K+

- Potassium is a major intracellular cation, with a positive charge.
- Potassium plays a major role in
  - Neuromuscular functions
    - Normal muscle functions that help us sit, walk or even breathe.
  - Cardiac functions
    - Contractions of the heart and regularity of its rhythm.
  - Acid-Base balance
  - Carbohydrate metabolism
  - Protein synthesis
  - Enzyme action.
- Potassium amounts to 43mmol per kg body weight.
- Percentage found in extracellular fluids is 2%.

- Usual dietary intake of potassium, is between 1500–4700 mg (40–120mmol) per day.
- Minimum requirement is between 1600–2000 mg (40–50mmol) per day.
- All the dietary potassium – whatever the food source – is absorbed in the upper gastrointestinal tract.
- Excretion of potassium is mainly through the renal system – urine and minor losses through faeces and sweat.

Thus, it becomes utmost important for Chronic Kidney Disease patients to be vigilant about their dietary potassium intake.

The normal range of potassium in our blood (serum) is 3.5 to 4.5 meq per litre.

Rise in serum potassium levels, above the normal range, it is known as **Hyperkalemia**.

Hyperkalemia may occur due to:

1. Increased dietary potassium intake in the presence of renal dysfunction.
2. Shift of potassium from inside of the cells (intracellular) to the fluids outside the cells (extracellular). This shift may occur with metabolic acidosis, hemolysis (breakdown of blood cells, which releases potassium from inside the cells into the blood circulation) and Rhabdomyolysis (breakdown of skeletal muscle cells).
3. Impaired renal excretion of potassium in cases of renal failure.

4. ACE inhibitors: An angiotensin-converting-enzyme-inhibitor (ACE-inhibitor) is a pharmaceutical drug used primarily for the treatment of hypertension and congestive heart failure. Examples are Captopril, Enalapril, Lisinopril. Most common side effect of these medications is hyperkalaemia.

Decrease in serum potassium levels, below the normal range, it is known as **hypokalemia**.

Hypokalemia may occur due to:

1. Diuretic medications are also called as Water Pills. They cause increase in potassium loss through the urine. This results in decreased potassium in the blood..
2. Anti-fungal medications like Amphotericin B. The binding of Amphotericin B to renal tubular collecting duct cells causes the leakage of potassium with resultant Hypokalemia.
3. Steroid excess conditions like Cushing's syndrome, Aldosteronism, Exogenous steroid use.
4. Gastro-intestinal losses during diarrhoea.
5. Renal Tubular Acidosis, a condition in which potassium is lost in the urine.

Severe Hypokalemia or Hyperkalemia may cause life threatening problems including abnormal heart rhythm and severe muscle weakness.

Majority of the potassium in blood comes from our diet.

Thus, dietary factors should be regulated to keep the vital K+ in check.

Our Indian diet includes:

- Carbohydrates as in *roti*, rice, *bhakri, naan*.
- Proteins as in *dals*, sprouts, milk, curds, *paneer* and in non-vegetarian sources as in eggs, meat, fish.
- Fats as in oils and ghee.
- Vegetables.
- Fruits.

Everything that is living, that we consume, has potassium in it. So, when we eat meat, we are consuming potassium as well.

Proteins are needed to maintain our nutrition and calorie balance.

Proteins in the diet, should be in the right amounts to give enough nourishment and at the same time, avoid excess potassium supply.

Hence, the right quality and quantity of nutrients need to be taken in our daily diet.

Certain foods are rich in potassium (more than 200 mg), some have moderate potassium (between 100 to 200 mg) and few are low in potassium levels (up to 100 mg per 100 gm of serving size).

In CKD, there is a big no-no to high potassium foods, moderate potassium foods are allowed in strictly limited quantities and the low potassium level foods are allowed in sufficient quantities.

The list is as follows:

1. **High Potassium Foods**

    a. Cereals: *Bajra*
    b. Pulses: *Arhar dal* or *Tuvar dal, Moong dal, Chana dal, Udad dal, Masur dal.*
    c. Sprouts, whole *moong*, whole *chana*, black *chana, rajma, chhole, barbati, maa ki dal* (whole *masur*), whole *udad*.
    d. Dried fruits and nuts like almonds, cashews, dates, raisins, figs *(anjeer)*, walnuts, pistachios etc.
    e. Fruits: Mango, banana, *chikoo (sapota)*, sweet lime *(mosambi)*, grapes, cherries, berries, peach, muskmelons.
    f. Vegetables: All green leafy vegetables. Root vegetables as potato, sweet potato, yam *(suran)*, colocassia *(arvi)* and lotus stem *(kamal dandi)*.
    g. Spices: Cloves*(laung)*, Cinnamon*(dalchini)*, Peppers (black pepper-*kali miri*, red chilli peppers-*lal mirch*).
    h. Beverages: Coconut water, coffee, fruit juices, vegetable juices and soups, condensed milk, drinking chocolate, and hard drinks.
    i. Other items: Black salt, rock salt, *saindhav namak, sanchar namak,* low sodium salts, ice-creams.

2. **Moderate Potassium Foods**

    a. Cereals: Wheat, *maida, jowar*, corn.
    b. *Dals*: All deskinned and polished *dals* and lentils.
    c. Fruits: Peach, orange, watermelons.

d. Vegetables: Onion, radish, carrot, bitter gourds, brinjals, cabbage, cauliflower, lady's finger, ginger, tomatoes and beans.
   e. Spices: All spices in large quantities.
   f. Beverages: Cow's milk and its milk products.

3. Low Potassium Foods

   a. Cereals: Rice, *poha*, semolina, vari (*bhagar, sama chawal, upvaas ka chawal*), *sabudana*.
   b. Fruits: Guava, Apple, Pear, Papaya, Pineapple. (Quantity as specified by Renal nutritionist).
   c. Vegetables: Gourds, *lauki, kaddu,* cucumber, green beans, green peas, garlic.
   d. Beverages: Buffalo milk and its milk products.
   e. Other items: White vinegar, honey, dried ginger, mint.

For CKD, one would assume that the low potassium list is the best. However, there are disadvantages of sticking to just one list.

- Indian vegetarian diets require *dals,* lentils and pulses to fulfil the protein requirements even for kidney patients.
- If the patients are on haemodialysis, they already are losing some proteins in the form of amino acids through the process.
- Peritoneal dialysis also drains out 5–10 grams of protein every day.
- Variety and choices become limited. Patients start disliking foods.

All about Potassium

Way out-

Leaching: Leaching is a process of removal of the water-soluble elements from vegetables, *dals* and pulses.

This helps in:

- Reducing potassium from the vegetables, *dals* and pulses.
- Allowing variety of food items from medium potassium list to be included in our diet.
- Protecting our heart from the hazards of high potassium levels i.e. hyperkalaemia.

Leaching Process

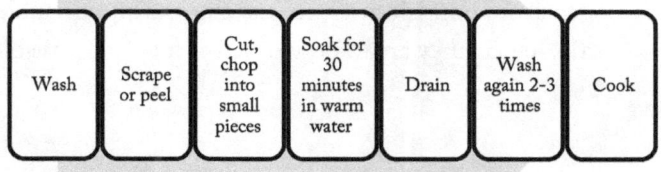

For vegetables

Vegetables

- Select low or medium potassium vegetable from the list given above.
- Wash the vegetable in room temperature water.
- Scrape or peel the vegetable, if possible.

- Cut the vegetable into small pieces, chop as small as possible.
- Soak this cut-chopped vegetable in plain, room temperature water or warm water. The water amount should be at least 10% more than the amount of vegetables. Optionally, add one tablespoon of white vinegar to it. Soak for a period of 30–45 minutes.
- Remember, if you are allergic to vinegar, do not add it for soaking vegetables.
- Drain the water. Wash the vegetable again in fresh water for 2–3 times.
- Cook in less oil or ghee, as required.
- No need to boil or pressure-cook the vegetables.
- This method should be useful on low or medium potassium containing fruit-vegetables.
- Green leafy vegetables and root vegetables do not leach out potassium as much as the routine vegetables do, hence, they are to be avoided as much as possible.

Dals

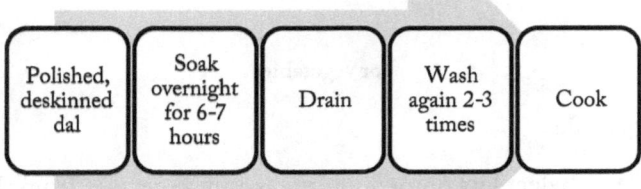

For dals/ lentils

- Preferably use polished, de-skinned *dals*.
- Soak raw *dal*, as much required for the whole family, in room temperature water, for 6–7 hours or overnight.
- In the morning, or after 7 hours, drain the water, wash the *dal* again in water for 2–3 times, and then directly cook in the pressure cooker.
- No need to discard the water after pressure cooking the *dal*.
- If you have forgotten to soak the raw *dal* overnight, then soak the *dal* in boiling hot water for 30–60 minutes, then drain the water and again wash for 2–3 times before pressure cooking.

Pulses and Sprouts

- *Moth, moong, barbati*, green peas (fresh and dried) and yellow peas are allowed.
- *Rajma*, black gram, *chana*, whole *udad*, whole *masur*, *chole* and *kadve waal* are to be strictly avoided.
- In case of *moth and moong*, they should be sprouted, then boiled in water for 10 minutes, their skins and water should be separated and the patient should have only the naked, sprouted seed. Alternatively, these can also be pressure-cooked till one whistle, on low flame, with some extra water added. This excess water, along with the skins should be separated from the sprouts.
- In case of peas and *barbarti*, they should be soaked overnight, pressure cooked till two whistles, on low flame, with excess water. Now, separate the excess water and then use the seeds.

Please note, not all of the potassium can be removed or leached out by this process. Hence, it is best to avoid high potassium foods and stick to the renal diet.

Please remember, these steps can be followed for cooking of the whole family's diet, so that the patient feels included.

- If we are leaching for everyone, then what about the potassium intake of the rest of the family members?

Well, the family members can always have dried fruits and nuts, lime juice, fresh fruits and juices, coconut water, *amla* and green leafy vegetables, to make up for the potassium, if required.

- What about other nutrient losses due to leaching?

Yes, along with potassium, vital water- soluble vitamins and nutrients are also lost. Kindly take prescribed vitamins from your Nephrologist.

Points to Remember

- ✓ **Hyperkalaemia – increased blood potassium levels- is dangerous.**
- ✓ **Hypokalemia – decreased blood potassium levels – is dangerous.**
- ✓ **Maintain diet with potassium restriction.**
- ✓ **Follow the process of leaching.**
- ✓ **Moderation is the rule. Even low potassium foods, when taken in large amounts, may accumulate potassium, leading to high potassium levels.**

Chapter 10

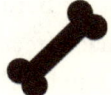

Phosphorus Care

Phosphorus and Calcium in our body are useful for

- The development of bones in our body,
- Their strength and
- Their sustainability.

Also, phosphorus is an essential component of Adenosine Triphosphate (ATP), which basically is the fuel that helps muscles contract and also runs a number of chemical reactions essential for life. The only source of phosphorus is the food that we eat. Whatever has protein, has phosphorus in it. So, beyond a point, we cannot reduce its intake. Excess phosphorus is removed from our blood via kidneys through the urine. Thus, the levels of phosphorus in our blood are maintained.

The normal range of **Serum Phosphorus is 2.5–4.5 mg dl.**

Calcium and phosphorus metabolism are interrelated. They are together in the formation of bones.

In Chronic Kidney Disease, excess phosphorus remains in the blood as the failing kidneys are not efficient in its excretion. Thus, the levels of Serum Phosphorus rise. This leads to a lot of abnormal effects. Parathyroid Hormone (PTH) release is stimulated. This causes extraction of calcium from the bones and leads to weakness in the bones. Vitamin D formation is suppressed. So new bone formation is also halted. Extreme effect of this is osteomalacia – severely weak and painful bones.

Elevated Serum Phosphorus levels lead to symptoms such as:

- Irritation and itching
- Weakness in bones and muscles
- Pain in bones and joints
- Osteomalacia sometimes may lead to fractures following minor injuries.

Thus, the phosphorus in our diet needs to be kept within normal range.

Phosphorus is a mineral present in almost all food items. The foods that are rich in proteins are rich sources of phosphorus also.

There are two ways of dealing with the elevated Serum Phosphorus levels;

- **Medicines**
  - ➢ Consult the nephrologist about the symptoms of elevated phosphorus levels.

- ➢ Your routine blood tests would reveal the elevated levels.
- ➢ Phosphate binders are prescribed.
- ➢ This medicine attaches to the phosphorus coming from the food inside our intestines, hence the name.
- ➢ It helps reduce the phosphorus absorption and therefore prevent all the ill effects mentioned above.

- **Diet**
  - ➢ Protein sources need to be carefully chosen. Choose curds, cow's milk, soymilk, tofu and low-fat paneer.
  - ➢ Avoid root vegetables as carrot, radish, beet.
  - ➢ Avoid wheat items, use rice and maida instead.
  - ➢ Avoid green leafy vegetables, potatoes, sweet potatoes.
  - ➢ Avoid chocolates, dried fruits and nuts, peanuts, ice-creams, cold drinks and beverages.

Remember, phosphorus cannot be reduced by the process of leaching or boiling.

Thus, the phosphorus rich foods are to be cautiously, sparingly and judiciously consumed.

Chapter 11

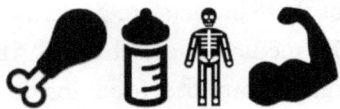

Proteins

- Building blocks of our body.
- Useful for growth and development.
- Supply amino acids.

Proteins are broadly classified into:

1. **First class proteins:** These are the high biological value proteins.

Biological Value is an index of protein quality that reflects the percentage of absorbed nitrogen from dietary protein retained by the body.

In simple words, biological value is a measure of the proportion of absorbed protein from a source. Higher the biological value, better is the amount of protein absorbed. This absorbed protein is easily available and becomes ready to form our body tissues.

They are the proteins that are entirely converted to amino acids after digestion.

Amino acids are the structural blocks of any protein.

This means these proteins are fully utilized for what they are known for, the building blocks of muscles and tissues- amino acids.

High Biological value proteins are mostly obtained from animal sources.

Egg is considered as the reference protein of first-class variety.

For example:

- Poultry,
- Lean meat,
- Fish,
- Egg whites,
- Milk and milk products as curds, buttermilk, *khoa*, cheese, *paneer*, *chhenna*, cottage cheese.

Soyabean when defatted i.e. the chunks or granules, is the only vegetarian protein source of high biological value.

2. **Second class proteins:** These are low biological value proteins.

They are proteins that are not entirely converted to amino acids after digestion.

They are obtained from plant sources, the leguminous variety, rich in nitrogen obtained from the soil.

For example:

- Dals,
- Pulses and
- Sprouts.

Apart from proteins, these plant sources give us carbohydrates, fats, fibre and minerals.

3. **Soya, a good vegetarian protein:** Soya protein is a plant source. Its biological value is near that of an egg.

Defatted soya chunks are the power houses of proteins.

One must be sure that one is not allergic to soy protein. Some Indians are allergic to soy.

Reference protein is a theoretical concept of the 'perfect protein' which is used with 100% efficiency at whatever level it is fed in the diet.

The term is used as a means of recommended intakes.

The nearest to this theoretical concept is the Egg protein.

So, Egg is the reference protein. Every other protein is compared to this reference protein.

Thus, soya converts biologically into good amount of protein after digestion.

Defatted soya chunks or granules should be used.

Refined soybean oil has no protein.

Amino Acids

The building blocks in proteins are called the **amino acids.**

The amino acids can be classified into essential and non-essential amino acids.

Essential Amino Acids

- Amino acids which need to be consumed in our daily diet are the essential amino acids.
- They cannot be synthesized in our body system and hence, need to be supplemented through diet.
- They are Valine, Leucine, Isoleucine, Threonine, Methionine, Phenylalanine, Lysine, Tryptophan and Histidine.

Non-essential Amino Acids

- By the nomenclature, they are not to be essentially eaten in our daily diet.
- This is because these amino acids can be synthesized in our body.
- They are Alanine, Serine, Cysteine, Aspartic acid, Glutamic acid and Hydroxyproline.

Conditionally Essential Amino Acids

As the name suggests, there are either specific dietary or host conditions under which functions are best maintained or improved when these amino acids are part of the nutrient intake.

Let's get back to Eating!

For CKD patients on conservative management, protein consumption needs to be at least **0.8 gm/ kg body weight/day**.

Various surveys have concluded that, the Indian diet, may it be vegetarian or even inclusive of non-vegetarian foods, does not meet the minimum requirement of protein on a daily basis.

Routine Indian pure vegetarian diet meets protein up to **0.3–0.6 gm/kg body weight/day**.

Routine Indian diet with non-vegetarian foods meets up to **0.4–0.8 gm/kg body weight/day.**

Certain Myths Prevail in Our Society

- Severe protein restrictions need to be followed in kidney disease patients.
- Zero protein diet will prevent further kidney damage.
- *Dals*, pulses, milk and milk products, eggs and non-vegetarian items need to be avoided in a kidney patient's diet.

As I said, these are myths. We need a minimum amount of protein intake to keep us healthy even if we are suffering from Chronic Kidney Disease.

Why?

- Protein is required for normal body building activities.
- Even in a fully grown adult, protein is required to rebuild the worn and torn tissues of vital body organs and muscles.

- Proteins help to maintain the original structure and functioning of our vital body organs for a long time.
- Proteins in the form of Albumin and Globulin are circulating in the blood. To maintain their blood levels and eventually blood balance, protein is required.
- Now, in case we follow the above prevalent "myths" and go on a very low protein or a zero-protein diet, the body building activities or the repair would not happen.
- Also, blood levels of protein would fall, leading to imbalance and swelling due to water retention.

The Consequences of Protein Deficiency are

- In children, growth is retarded.
- In adults, there is weight loss and loss of immunity.
- Haemoglobin formation is hampered with, resulting in anaemia. In CKD, the kidneys fail to form the hormone Erythropoietin, which is responsible for formation of haemoglobin in blood. On top of it, protein deficiency might contribute to further reduction of haemoglobin formation. Thus, protein intake needs to be adequately maintained.
- Prolonged deficiency may lead to inadequate synthesis of Plasma proteins- the Albumin and Fibrinogen.
    - Albumin deficiency – in severe stages- leads to swelling all over the body, oedema. Increased incidences of shock may occur.

- Fibrinogen deficiency may lead to bleeding disorder.
- Wound healing becomes delayed due to lack of proteins.
- Antibodies, which fight against infections, are made of proteins. Thus, our immunity, the capacity to fight infections, is reduced in case of protein deficiencies.
- Hormones are made of proteins. Severe protein deficiency may lead to hormonal imbalances.

There may be times when due to inadequate calorie-protein intake, **protein energy malnutrition** sets in. The body starts utilizing our own proteins from the muscles and eventually from the structure of vital body organs. This may lead to further weakness and damage to our internal organs.

So, eating adequate proteins is very important.

So, where has this concept of protein restriction for CKD diet come from?

The Western Diet Data

We come across the western diet data analysis, which enforces on restricted protein intakes in early stages of CKD.

But then looking into the western diets show a lot of meat intake, which may cause overload on the failing kidneys. They often cross the upper limit of 0.8 g/kg/day for proteins. So, those who cross this upper limit, need to be brought 'under' 0.8 g/kg/day and told to 'restrict' protein intake.

Indian diets per se, even if non-vegetarian foods are consumed (which is most often NOT daily), predominantly include second class proteins like dals, pulses, sprouts.

Our intakes do not cross borders of overload; rather they are on the lower side of the protein range. In fact, if they are found to be very low on calculations (e.g. 0.5 g/kg/day), the dietician needs to tell these CKD patients to actually increase protein content in the diet!

So, need not worry Indians!

Follow a proper diet under the guidance of an expert renal nutritionist.

The diet of a CKD patient requires 50% of proteins from first class sources and the other half from the second-class sources.

In case of pure vegetarians or vegans, plant-based protein nutrition needs to be calculated keeping in mind the potassium and phosphorus in the foods.

In case of patients on keto-analogue medications, a very low protein diet is advised, depending on the amount of medication prescribed. In this case, the amino acids are obtained through the keto-analogue medications.

In CKD Stage 1–4, the protein requirements are 0.8 gm per kg body weight per day and are calculated taking into consideration:

- Weight
- Age

- GFR
- Activity pattern
- Lifestyle
- Other pre-existing illnesses like Diabetes, Hypertension, Coronary events and status of nutrition.

For assessing the patients whether they are eating adequate proteins and calories, certain tools and techniques are used as Subjective Global Assessment (SGA) and Malnutrition Inflammation Score (MIS).

When proteins are consumed less, we tend to consume either more of carbohydrates or more of fats. Increase in fat intake increases the lipids in our blood.

Increase in carbohydrates leads to increased blood sugar levels. Apart from glycogen, excess calories from carbohydrates are also converted and stored in the form of fats and thus, again fat derangements occur. Obesity has its own triggers to the lipid cycle. The result is increased low density lipoproteins (LDL), cholesterols etc.

Thus, a balanced meal is advisable with proper guidance about each nutrient.

For example:

50 kg male, CKD stage 1–4, should consume 0.8 gm/kg/day of proteins that is

0.8 × 50 = 40 gm of proteins per day, out of which 20 gm should come from first class sources.

20 gm first class sources approximately include:

- 2 egg whites = 6 gm
- 300 ml of cow's milk = 6.6 gm
- 200 ml of cow milk curds = 4.4 gm
- 50 gm of paneer = 3 gm.

20 gm of second-class proteins approximately includes:

- 60 gm of raw *dal*, consumed after cooking, which amounts to 4 *katoris* of cooked, thick *dal* = 14 gm
- 10 gm of raw sprouts, consumed after sprouting and cooking = 2.3 gm
- 4 *phulkas*, each of 20 gm of wheat flour each = 6.4 gm

So, it is evident from the above exhaustive discussion, that *dals* and other protein sources should not be discarded from the diet. They actually need to be tailored by an expert in kidney diets.

Points to Remember

- ✓ **Protein restriction in the diet may lead to malnutrition and further worsening of CKD.**
- ✓ **A daily dietary intake of 0.8 gm per kilogram body weight per day of proteins must be consumed.**
- ✓ **Follow dietary advice for calculated protein intake.**
- ✓ **Remember, all the protein in our body either comes from the diet or from breaking down from our body organs to maintain blood levels and**

calories. Better to supply it through diet than from our internal organs.
- ✓ Indian diets contain a variety of proteins which are kidney friendly.

Chapter 12

Carbohydrates

Carbohydrates are:

- Found in basic food sources in our daily diet.
- Main source of energy.
- Staple diet. Means without them, our diet is not complete.
- Economical and easily available energy source.
- **55%–60%** of the total diet. Same should be in CKD diet as well.

Carbohydrate-rich food items in our diet are:

- Rice
- Wheat
- *Poha*
- *Rawa*
- *Seviya*
- *Maida*
- *Jowar*
- *Bajra*
- Maize

- *Nachni* (ragi)
- Potatoes, sweet potatoes, colocassia (*arvi*), yam (*suran*), beetroot,
- Sago (*sabudana*),
- *Vari* (*samachawal*) and
- All fruits

Our routine diet consists of three major sources of carbohydrates:

1. Sucrose or cane sugar or simple sugar or jaggery,
2. Lactose, which is present in milk,
3. Starches, which are present in all food grains.

Process of Carbohydrate Digestion

- When we eat, we take small morsels and chew.
- The more, the slower and the longer we chew, more and more forms the saliva (the secretions of the mouth) that gets mixed with food.
- This saliva breaks down the carbohydrate molecules into digestible forms.
- **Carbohydrate digestion starts in the mouth. Eat slow, chew properly. Do not eat in a hurry.**
- Later when we swallow food, our stomach mixes carbohydrates.
- Small intestine further breaks it down and simple forms are ready for getting absorbed in the blood.

Absorption of carbohydrates takes place in the form of glucose directly into the blood stream.

Glucose is the final digestion product of our most abundant carbohydrate food, the starches.

Now we know the importance of chewing food '32' times as told by our elders. We should eat slow so that the saliva is well mixed with food. Now we are aware that the carbohydrate digestion starts in the mouth itself.

Categorization of carbohydrates, according to the amount of potassium present in them per 100 gm is as follows:

1. **Freely allowed:** Can be used daily in prescribed amounts.

    - Rice,
    - Wheat,
    - *Maida* (refined flour)
    - Sago (*sabudana*),
    - *Sama* (*vari or bhagar*),
    - *Poha*
    - Semolina *(rawa).*

2. **Moderate use:** Can be used once in a week.

    - Jowar,
    - *Seviya* and
    - *Jaada poha*

3. **Restricted use:** Can be used once in a month. Consume in moderate amounts.

    - Bajra,
    - Maize
    - *Nachni* (ragi).

Daily Treats

- Rice, *pulavs*, *masale bhaat*, curd rice, *bisibele bhaat*, *Pongal*,
- Rotis, *phulkas*, *chapatis*, plain *paratha*, *puris*, *bhakris*, *bhaturas*, *naans*, *baatis*, *baflas*,
- *Sabudana khichdi*, *sabudana thalipeeth*, *sabudana vadas*,
- *Samachawal for upawas*,
- *Patla poha* with vegetables,
- *Upma* with vegetables,
- *Idlis*, made of rice or *rawa*, *dosas*, *uttapams* and
- Sometimes bread can be in the menu planning. (Remember, anything in excess is dangerous, even if it is in the "allowed" category).

Cornflakes and oats are processed, so need to be avoided as far as possible.

Eat freshly cooked foods to retain their nutrients or within three hours of cooking.

Weekend Treats

- *Jowar ki roti*,
- *Seviya ki kheer* or *seviya upma*
- *Poha* with vegetables or *dadpe pohe* (Konkani)

Avoid, as Much as Possible

- *Bajre ki roti* or *bhakri*,
- *Bhuttas* and corns
- *Nachni (ragi) sheera* or *bhakri*.

These are restricted due to high potassium levels.

Chapter 13

Fats

Fats are the oils and ghee which we use for cooking.

Some fats are also present in invisible or dissolved forms in many food items. They are present in nuts, oil seeds, milk, butter, in eggs as cholesterol, in fishes and in and around the meat we consume.

Why are fats essential for our body?

- Fats supply energy,
- Protect vital body organs by making a cushion-like layer around them,
- Carry fat soluble vitamins A, D, E & K.
- They add flavour to our food.
- They add satiety, means give a sense of satisfaction after eating.

Fats form the third major nutrient of the food we consume, the other two being carbohydrates and proteins.

There are two types of fats, according to their chemical composition:

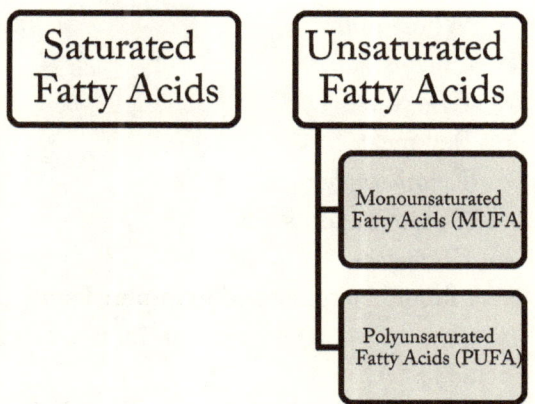

Types of Fats

1. Saturated Fatty Acids (SFA)
2. Unsaturated Fatty Acids (UFA). These again are of two types the Poly-Unsaturated Fatty Acids – the PUFA and the Mono-Unsaturated Fatty Acids – the MUFA.

Saturated Fatty Acids

- The fats which turn into solid, thick state from their liquid state are the saturated fatty acids.
- They turn solids when the temperature is cold. During summers and if heated, they turn back into liquid state.
- SFA are found in animal products such as
  - Butter
  - Ghee
  - Cream

- Whole milk
- Cheese, *Paneer*
- Egg-yolk
- Red meat
- *Vanaspati ghee*
- Coconut and its oils
- Chocolates.

- SFA should be consumed in minimal amounts.
- 10% of the total fat content in the diet should include SFA.
- SFA rich diet tends to increase blood cholesterol. But they are essential as Medium chain triglycerides.

Unsaturated Fatty Acids

- Mainly found in plant-based oils.
- These are chemically classified as PUFA and MUFA.
- This PUFA – MUFA are present in a combined state in the oils.
- Every vegetable oil has PUFA-MUFA in it, in a specific percentage.
- This makes them either PUFA-rich or MUFA-rich oils.
- Both oils have their own advantages in terms of heart health.

For example: Oils from

- Sunflower seeds
- Safflower seeds
- Cotton seeds

- Sesame seeds
- Mustard seeds
- Soybeans
- Groundnuts
- Corn
- Olives
- Almonds
- Rice bran
- Fish

Unsaturated fatty acids should comprise about **25%** of the total fat requirements in a CKD diet.

Trans – Fats

Trans fats are basically artificial fats.

They are formed artificially by hydrogenation of vegetable oils. In this process, the vegetable oils are turned into solid state from their free-flowing, liquid nature. Hydrogenation has seen to be of major use in food industry, as it improves the shelf-life of the oils, as well as add to the taste and crispiness of the food item in which it is used.

Examples of trans fats (TFA) are the *Vanaspathi* oils (the solid *Dalda* as we know from old days) sold as Vegetable ghee in the market.

Naturally occurring TFAs are found in small amounts in meat and dairy products. Their health effects are being studied yet.

Effects of TFAs on Our Body

- TFAs are found to be a greater risk for Chronic Degenerative Diseases like Alzheimers, Parkinsons, Dementia, Spinal muscular atrophy, cancers, cystic fibrosis etc.
- TFAs are more atherogenic than saturated fatty acids. Atherogenesis means the accumulation and deposition of fatty deposits in the arteries.
- TFAs increase the bad cholesterols and reduce the amount of good- HDL cholesterol in blood.
- TFAs increase the abnormal clotting of blood.
- **Studies show the relation of TFAs and cancers and Diabetes.**

Following are some ways to avoid the TFA intake in our diet:

- Avoid bakery products as chips, cookies, cakes and pastries.
- Cook using cold pressed oils as mustard, olive, sesame oils.
- Avoid using hydrogenated vegetable oils, *vanaspathi* ghee and margarines.
- Avoid using Vegetable butter, marketed as low cholesterol, low fat butter. It is same as TFAs. Use normal, routine butter instead.
- Do not heat oil for a long time for cooking or frying.

- Do not reuse the oil left after frying or cooking.
- Avoid reheating of oils.
- Avoid mixing of two different oils or oil and ghee in the same cooking vessel. Different oils have different boiling points and mixing them may prove hazardous combination for our heart and blood vessels.
- Check nutrition labels on packaged foods as Margarine, shortening, vegetable ghee, partially hydrogenated vegetable oils, or low fat, low cholesterol butter. They are all TFAs.

Chapter 14

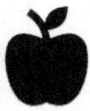

Fruits

Fruits are Classified as

Fresh fruits and Dried fruits.

1. Dried Fruits and Nuts

- The dried, dehydrated, desiccated fruits are rich sources of vitamins and minerals especially potassium.
- In CKD, the failing kidneys are not able to excrete the excess of potassium through the urine.
- It is better to avoid the consumption of dried fruits and nuts for that matter, to protect the kidneys as much as possible.

2. Fresh Fruits

- Fresh fruits are also rich in potassium.
- There are Low, Medium and High potassium containing fruits.

- The low potassium containing fruits are allowed in case of CKD patients with controlled blood potassium levels.
- Remember, any low potassium source taken in excess amounts than prescribed, turns into a medium or high potassium source for patients.
- Thus, moderation and following the prescription is the key to healthy eating habits and healthy lifestyle.

List of Low Potassium fruits allowed in prescribed amounts in CKD patients:

- Guava
- Apple
- Pear
- Pineapple
- Papaya
- Orange
- Green Mango

All the other fruits should be consumed only under the guidance of your Nephrologist and renal dietitian.

Lift up your spirits everyone!

Fruits can be turned into some exotic, mouth-watering, delicious bites!

- **Fruit Ice:** Chop some fruit, fill it into trays or kulfi-makers and put them into the freezer compartment. Relish delicious fruit ice whenever required.
- **Frozen fruits:** Chunks of peeled fruits can be frozen and relished in summers to quench thirst.

This helps to reduce the water intake and prevents swelling.
- **Flavored yogurts:** Chop some fruit into low-fat yogurt, refrigerate if you like it cold and relish it as ice-creams.
- **Frozen flavored *Kheers* and *Basundi* and *Rabadi:*** Milk and chopped fruits and jaggery and refrigerate.
- **Arrow-root jelly with fruits:** Cook and cool arrowroot (arrow-root flour is low in potassium), cool it into a nice-shaped mold to form a jelly. Add chopped fruits as toppings or add chopped fruits while pouring the mixture into the mold.

Relish fruits - follow the rule of moderation and be happy!

Remember:

GAP3- Guava, Apple, Pear, Pineapple, Papaya

Chapter 15

Vegetables

Vegetables are an integral part of Indian diet. Without vegetables, our plate looks incomplete, our tummies feel not full and the wholesomeness in our diet suffers.

Thus, vegetables are a must in our daily diet. They may be eaten:

- Cooked as in the form of vegetables and soups
- Raw in the form of salads
- In the mixed forms as in *kachumbers*, *raitas* and all kinds of chopped, grated, crushed and pickled forms.

Out of the above options, soups and pickled forms of vegetables are to be restricted in the diet of CKD patients.

Rest all the forms of vegetables is welcome.

Remember: From Chapter9 – All About Potassium:
Leaching Process:
Vegetables:

- *Select low or medium potassium vegetable from the list given below.*
- *Wash the vegetable in room temperature water.*
- *Scrape or peel the vegetable, if possible.*
- *Cut the vegetable into small pieces, chop as small as possible.*
- *Soak this cut-chopped vegetable in plain warm water, at least 10% more than the amount of vegetables. Add one tablespoon of white vinegar to it. Soak for a period of 30–45 minutes.*
- *Remember, if you are allergic to vinegar, do not add it for soaking vegetables.*
- *Drain the water, wash the vegetable again in fresh water for 2–3 times.*
- *Cook in less oil or ghee, as required.*
- *No need to boil or pressure-cook the vegetables.*
- *This method should be useful on low or medium potassium containing fruit-vegetables or other vegetables.*
- *Green leafy vegetables and root vegetables do not leach out potassium as much as the routine vegetables do, hence, they should be avoided as much as possible.*

The wide range of vegetables available in Indian markets can be categorically placed under four broad heads:

1. Root Vegetables

a. Potato
b. Sweet potato
c. Yam (*Suran*)
d. Colocassia *(Arvi)*

e. Lotus stem (*kamal kakdi or kamal ki dandi*)
   f. Beet
   g. Radish
   h. Carrot
   i. Tapioca

Out of this list, the vegetables that can be consumed by CKD patients, non-diabetic, are Radish and Carrot.

The rest of the vegetables from this list need to be restricted for consumption, once in a month, in smaller quantities.

This is due to the high potassium and mineral content of these vegetables.

Remember, restrictions are to prevent the burden of potassium overload in the blood.

Moderation is the Rule!

2. Green Leafy Vegetables

   a. *Agathi* leaves (a type of Spinach)
   b. Amaranth leaves, green *(Rajgira* leaves, green in colour)
   c. Amaranth leaves, red (*Rajgira* leaves, red in colour)
   d. Basella leaves (Indian spinach, Malabar spinach)
   e. *Bathua* leaves
   f. Beet greens
   g. Betel leaves (*Paan*)
   h. Brussels sprouts (type of small cabbage, same family)
   i. Chinese cabbage

j. Cabbage, green, violet,
k. Cauliflower leaves
l. Colocasia leaves *(Arvi* leaves)
m. Drumstick leaves
n. *Dil* leaves *(Sua saag)*
o. Fenugreek leaves (*methi)*
p. Garden cress (*Halim* leaves)
q. *Gogu* leaves, green and red *(Gongura* leaves)
r. *Knol-khol* leaves
s. Lettuce leaves (salad leaves)
t. Mustard leaves (*sarson*)
u. Pak Choi leaves (type of cabbage leaves, found across Asia)
v. Parsley (*Ajmoda, ajwain*)
w. *Ponnaganni* (Koypa leaves, found in water)
x. Pumpkin leaves
y. Radish leaves
z. Spinach
aa. Tamarind leaves

The long list of green leafy vegetables, available in India, suggests the rich heritage of our food culture.

Green leaves are rich sources of potassium.

After cooking, the quantity of the cooked vegetable becomes less and thus, large amounts of the leaves are required, in weight.

This may lead to consumption of large amounts of mineral-rich, especially potassium-rich vegetables.

Thus, **restriction** is a must here.

Vegetables

Spinach (palak) and fenugreek (*methi*) are frequently in question, so these vegetables are allowed once in a month and in combination with other vegetables and in moderate quantities.

Remember, **moderation is the key**!

3. **Other Vegetables or Fruit Vegetables**
    a. Ash gourd (white pumpkin, *petha*)
    b. Bitter gourd (*karela*)
    c. Bottle gourd (*lauki)*
    d. Brinjal, all varieties
    e. Broad beans *(Sem phalli)*
    f. Capsicum, green, red and yellow
    g. Cauliflower
    h. Celery stalk (*Ajwain ki dandi)*
    i. Chow-chow (type of vegetable-pear)
    j. Cluster beans (*guar phalli)*
    k. Colocasia stem, black and green (*Taro ki dandi)*
    l. Corn
    m. Cucumber, all types
    n. Drumsticks
    o. Field beans (*Vaal phalli)*
    p. French beans, green and violet *(Shravan Ghevada)*
    q. Jack fruit *(Phanas)*
    r. Knol-khol or Naval kaval
    s. *Kovai*, big and small (*Tendli/ Kundru*)
    t. Ladies finger/ Okra/ *Bhindi*
    u. Mango, raw, green
    v. Onions
    w. Garlic

- x. Ginger
- y. Chillies
- z. Papaya, raw
- aa. *Parwar*
- ab. Green peas, fresh
- ac. Green plantain (Green banana)
- ad. Pumpkin, green, orange
- ae. Ridge gourd (*Dodka*)
- af. Snake gourd *(Parwal)*
- ag. *Tinda/Dhemus*
- ah. Tomato, green and red
- ai. Zucchini (*Turai)*
- aj. Mushrooms

The process of leaching on the above "Other vegetables" removes maximum amount of potassium from them.

Thus, these are the vegetables which should be consumed on a regular basis by all CKD patients.

The list is large, variety is assured, and taste is guaranteed after leaching.

And no boiling of the vegetables or pressure cooking them in large amounts of water is required.

Exceptions are always part of this world, and here, it is

- Tomatoes
- Plantain greens and
- Raw jackfruit.

Culinary skills back into action now! Thanks Ma!

Vegetables

Cooking requires:

- Oil or ghee (discussed in Chapter 13 – Fats)
- Salt (discussed in Chapter 8 – Salt and Sodium)
- Sugar (sometimes. Please used white, refined sugar or jaggery. Sugar-like substances, marketed as sugar-substitutes, low or zero in calories are in fact "Chemicals". Kidney patients and all others need to be aware and beware of chemicals entering our body. Unknowingly or knowingly, many chemicals enter our body through various food items. These are thrown out or excreted from our body through kidneys as urine, travel through liver or come out through sweat, so why risk ourselves).
- Condiments and Spices, commonly known as the *tadka* and *masalas*.

Condiments and spices include:

- Mustard seeds (*Rai / Sarson*)
- Cumin seeds *(Jeera)*
- Sesame seeds (*til*)
- Carom seeds/ Thymol/ Celery seeds/ *Ajwain*
- Poppy seeds (*Khaskhas*)
- Fenugreek seeds *(methi dana)*
- Coriander seeds (*sabut dhaniya, khada dhaniya, dhane)*
- Pomegranate seeds *(Anardana)*
- Turmeric *(Haldi)*
- Chillies, red, powdered or green
- Dry mango powder *(amchoor)*
- Cloves (*Laung*)

- Black pepper (*kali mirch, kali miri*)
- Asafetida *(Hing)*
- Nutmeg *(Jaiphal)*
- Mace *(Javitri/Jaypatri)*
- Curry leaves (*Kadhi patta*)
- Chia seeds *(Sabza)*
- *Charoli (Chironji dana)*
- Coriander leaves
- Mint leaves *(Pudina)*
- Bay leaves *(Tejpatta)*
- *Kalpasi (Patthar ke phool)*
- Dry Ginger *(Sonth)*
- Cardamom (*Elaichi*, small and big)
- Cinnamon stick (*dalchini*)
- Caraway/ Nigella seeds *(Kalonji)*
- Star Anise (*Chakri phool*)
- Fennel seeds *(Saunf)*
- Saffron *(Kesar)*

These spices should be used in moderate quantities.

The **garam masala** or hot Indian spices category like cloves, black pepper, cinnamon and red chilly peppers should be avoided as far as possible.

Again, the question of potassium in these spices arises.

Potassium, in 100 grams of each of the listed condiments and spices is high.

But look at the amount we are using in our cuisines. When used in moderation and once in a week, theses spices can be used in the foods of CKD patients, to give them taste.

The list is large.

We do not use all the spices in a single recipe. Every recipe has a unique combination of spices.

Moderation is the way to go here, for a yummy, tasty meal on everyday basis.

Remember:

Certain recipes require nuts and dried fruits like almonds, cashews, pistachios, dried pumpkin seeds (*magaz bi*) and raisins, dates, dried dates and cream to make the gravies creamier, richer and smoother.

These nuts and dried fruits need to be avoided as much as possible. Alternative culinary options need to be chosen.

After all, Choice is Yours, as Life is Yours!

Remember: Leaching

Chapter 16

Food Items to Strictly Avoid – The Big No-No's

Foods items in CKD patients should be

- Cautiously selected
- Meticulously cooked
- Moderately consumed
- Satisfying the appetite.

CKD stage 1 to 4 are the conservative stages.

Here, the failing kidneys need to be protected from further damage by:

- Keeping blood pressure under control.
- Strict control on blood sugars and make sure they remain steady, no spikes of high or low sugars are acceptable.
- Infection control: Prevent outside eating, street foods, viral and bacterial infections by keeping excellent personal hygiene.

Food Items to Strictly Avoid – The Big No-No's

- Stress: Physical, mental and psychological stress should be kept to a minimum or avoided.
- Nutrition: Malnutrition needs to be prevented by following the Renal Dietary Guidelines and Exercise and Life-style pattern.

By adhering to the basics of preventive measures, the stages of CKD can be prolonged.

Though it differs from patient to patient as to how the CKD progression occurs, we can definitely keep ourselves nutritionally, physically and psychologically fit for our day-to-day activities and future.

Keeping Blood Pressure Under Control

- Use Common salt (Sodium chloride, sea-salt, refined, iodized).
- Measure salt daily and stick to the amounts.
- Avoid eating *papads, pickles, chutneys,* jams, sauces, wafers, ketchups, ready to eat items with preservatives, Chinese sauces, salted items like salted *chana* or peanuts or *kurmura*, items with artificial colors, processed vegetables or meat.
- Measure the amount of water to be consumed in a day.
- Discuss about salt and water with your nephrologist during every visit. Remember, blood and body parameters may change every time and so does fluid intake, salt intake and diet.

(Exceptions is the rule of life; thus, discussion brings light of knowledge!)

Strict control on blood sugars and make sure they remain steady, no spikes of high or low are acceptable:

- Complex carbohydrates such as whole grains, pulses and legumes should be consumed.
- Avoid refined, processed and ready to eat meals.
- Include fresh vegetables and fruits - that are allowed - in every meal.
- Adhere to meal timings. Do not skip meals.
- Watch for portion control. Anything in excess may disturb the sugar balance.
- Carb-counting should be adopted, if variety is on the menu. For example: If you feel like having an extra serving of plain garlic naan with tandoori *paneer*, for that meal, avoid eating rice completely. Replace one type of carbohydrate by another, keeping in mind the amount of serving and the fiber intake along with it.
- Avoid white, refined sugars and other chemicals which taste like sugars.
- Consume natural sweeteners.

Infection Control

- **Avoid outside eating,**
- **Street foods,**
- **Viral and bacterial infections by keeping excellent personal hygiene.**

This is to avoid extra burden on our body. Our body mechanisms are already fighting the imbalances due to the accumulation of metabolic wastes in our blood. Thus, our body needs to be protected from the external factors entering into it and causing disturbances.

Stress: Physical, mental and psychological stress should be kept to a minimum or avoided.

- Inculcate a healthy lifestyle.
- Quit smoking, drinking, chewing *paan* or tobacco or *gutkhas*.
- Fix meal timings and sleep timings.
- Schedule an early morning walk or yoga or light exercises with meditation on a daily basis. Exercise releases endorphins, which are happiness hormones. They refresh you for the whole day.
- Read books, listen to music, paint, have gardening activities, evening activities with family and friends, social work- any of this- even if you are a working person or businessperson.
- Perform Brain Gym activities like solving sudoku puzzles, mathematics puzzles, learning a new skill or a new musical instrument. Break the monotony in your life.

Nutrition: Malnutrition needs to be prevented by following the Renal Dietary Guidelines and Exercise and Life-style pattern.

- Be regular with your follow-ups with the Nephrologist and Renal nutritionist.
- Strictly adhere to the dietary guidelines.
- There are myths around the intake of Proteins, type of salt, cooking methods of vegetables etc. Kindly

discuss them appropriately before incorporating in the daily routine.
- Do not indulge into "Kidney – cleansing" or flushing medications, juices, *kadhas*, decoctions or anything that is given to you in the name of alternative medicines.
- Remember, the kidneys are structurally and functionally formed when the babies are in the mother's womb. Kidney tissues and structures are not reformed or repaired by anything. The structure of the kidney tissues and its functions age as we age. Thus, in case of CKD, which could be due to any reason, the kidneys need to be protected and prevented from further damage but cannot be reverted back to normal physically and functionally.

The Big No-No's

- **Aerated, carbonated beverages**, commonly known as Cold drinks. They contain preservatives and phosphoric acids, which is extremely harmful for the bones. They will add to phosphorus load which is difficult to remove with failing kidneys. Phosphorus is difficult to remove by dialysis as well.
- **Non-branded herbal or Chinese or green teas**, usually in powdered form. These may cause severe liver damage.
- **Tobacco** smoking or chewing.
- Strong coffee. **Coffee** has potassium in large amounts. It is preferable to drink coffee in small amounts with milk.

Food Items to Strictly Avoid – The Big No-No's

- **Black tea** or too long brewed tea without milk. This yields a lot of potassium. Also, the **lemon grass** in tea is a high source of potassium.
- **Coconut water** and **dried fruits** and **nuts** are to be avoided, because they too have concentrated form of potassium. Also, the artificial colors and gases used to dry them may contain large amounts of hidden sodium and chemicals harmful to the already failing kidneys.
- **Any ready to eat item** with labelled Class 2 or Class 3 preservatives.
- **Soy sauce**, used in Chinese menu, as well as **Ajinomoto**, which is again Monosodium glutamate, a chemical with sodium.
- **Processed meats and fishes.**
- **Processed cheese and hard-smoked cheese.**
- **Ready to eat vegetables.**
- **Bakery items.**
- **Chocolates.**
- **Canned** and **tinned foods.**
- **Rich gravies** with excess amounts of **dried fruits, spices and oil.**
- **Do not mix oil and ghee in the same container.** Do not heat them together. The ghee has a different heating point than that of oil. Thus, when mixed together for heating, one attains its boiling point, while the other is yet to. This may lead to the turning the earlier heated fat into a bad, rancid fat. This is extremely dangerous for the hearts and blood vessels. So, use oil and ghee separate. One Menu – One Fat (OMOF)!

Chapter 17

Kidney Disease Diets – Myths and Facts

Kidney disease, especially Chronic Kidney Disease is detected mostly in later stages in India. This is because of:

- Ignorance towards health and fitness.
- Uncontrolled diabetes
- Uncontrolled hypertension
- Lack of awareness about CKD of unknown origin.
- Delay in starting kidney treatment.
- Inability of patients in early stages of CKD to reach nephrologists.
- Trying out of alternative medicines, with the hope of complete recovery of kidneys.

Anatomically speaking, in fact, embryologically speaking, the kidneys are formed in the developmental stages of life, when we are in our mother's womb. Kidneys, once formed, start functioning intra-uterine.

It is like age. Our kidneys are the same age as we are, probably older, as they start functioning before we are even out in this world. They grow in the womb, start functioning and grow as we grow, age and grow old as we grow old.

Kidneys – once damaged – as in chronic kidney disease, do not structurally re-grow or are formed again. A bone may be repaired and grown, so is the skin and some other tissues. But vital organs like kidneys, heart, spleen, lungs do not structurally re-grow. They may, however, functionally grow stronger, enabling themselves to cope with the structurally damaged parts. This is exactly what happens in chronic diseases like CKD. The structural and functional unit in kidneys is the Nephron. Surviving nephrons take up the extra function of the failed nephrons of the kidneys. Which means, they have to do their own work and extra work as well to compensate for the loss of other nephrons. But how long can one sustain extra burden and overwork. Thus, work efficiency is hampered in the long run, the quality of work suffers and finally, the kidneys start showing the progression towards failure, that which we call the Stages of Chronic Kidney Disease. Measurement of serum Creatinine is a sensitive indicator of kidney functions. Estimation of Glomerular Filtration Rate, the eGFR, helps in establishing the work of kidneys considering the serum creatinine, age of the patient, sex and race.

This is the biggest myth we have as patients. The myth around this is- Kidneys can be completely revived, in case of CKD, back to their original structure and function, with the help of certain, alternative medications. However, the fact remains, that whatever the medicine or "pathy", the anatomy remains same and the fact remains the same that nephrons cannot be regenerated. New nephrons cannot be created by any external means.

Thus, all the patients diagnosed as CKD, need to follow the medicine and dietary guidelines.

Certain myths surround the renal diet.

Let us discuss them one by one, along with the facts.

1. Myth: Drink lots of water to flush our kidneys.

I will drink plenty of water to keep my kidneys normal. It will cure my kidney disease and if I don't have kidney disease, it will keep me away from it.

Fact:

For CKD patients, the 24-hour urine output plus 500 millilitres of plain water intake is sufficient to remove toxic wastes from our system.

Extra water, other than the required amount may cause "system overload" on the heart and the failing kidneys. Extra water gets accumulated in the ankles, feet and sometimes, when it exceeds, it takes the empty places in the abdominal cavity and the lungs, replacing the air in the lungs with fluid. This results in breathlessness and emergencies. Also, the heart needs to pump extra water throughout, continuously for 24 hours. This leads to over-working of the heart. Imagine the tired, fatigued heart! What if it gives way?

If your kidneys are normal, drinking excess water may prevent stone formation. However, it cannot prevent kidney failure that may happen because of diabetes, hypertension and glomerulonephritis.

2. Myth: We eat less salt daily.

So **we use other salts, which are "good salts".** Doctor told me low salt. I will use a low sodium salt. Its's the same thing!

Better still, I will use the natural *'sendha namak'*.

Fact:

Depending on the stage of CKD, the swelling (oedema) and the 24-hour urine output, 6–8 grams of common salt (free flow, refined, iodised, Sodium chloride, white salt) should be consumed. Properly measured amounts should be consumed daily.

Do we measure salt while eating?

Do we measure salt while cooking?

Do we have a separate, daily quota of salt and not use anything extra?

Which are the "Good salts"?

(Please refer to Chapter 8 – Salt and Sodium for detailed description).

3. Proteins in the diet of a Chronic Kidney Disease patient should be completely reduced or restricted or banned.

Fact:

Proteins in Indian diet are already on the lower limits of normal.

Kindly follow dietary guidelines, do not restrict proteins.

Follow the advice of expert nutritionists, who can help calculate your daily protein intake. Eat calculated and in moderation. Do not give up or give in too easily on your diet, medications and exercise. CKD in early cases can be controlled from further worsening or advancing, if and only if, the patients follow the medications, diet and exercise routine religiously. Blood pressures need to be kept under control, so are the blood sugars need to be prevented from frequent spikes of highs and lows.

If and only if the CKD stage 1 through 4 patient is on a Ketoanalogue diet, a special medication which is given to provide specific amino acids directly, bypassing the dietary whole proteins, then the patients need to follow a specific diet. This diet includes calculated amounts of proteins through diet and medication.

Otherwise, the required amount of proteins needs to be consumed.

Why is protein necessary?

If protein intake does not meet the immediate requirements in case of illness in CKD, the body repairing, and healing effects of proteins cannot be maintained at a required rate.

The consequences of protein deficiency are:

- In children, growth is retarded.
- In adults, there is weight loss.

- Haemoglobin information is hampered with consequent anaemia. In CKD, the kidneys gradually fail to form the hormone Erythropoietin, which is responsible for formation of haemoglobin in blood. On top of it, if protein deficiency contributes to further reduction of haemoglobin formation, then the crisis of lowered haemoglobin or anaemia is to be experienced in the earlier stages of CKD. Thus, protein intake needs to be adequately maintained.
- Prolonged deficiency may lead to inadequate synthesis of Plasma proteins- the Albumin and Fibrinogen.
  - Albumin deficiency – in severe stages- leads to swelling all over the body, oedema. Increased incidences of shock may occur.
  - Fibrinogen deficiency may lead to bleeding disorder.
- Wound healing becomes delayed due to lack of proteins.
- Antibodies, which fight against infections, are made of proteins. Thus, our immunity, the capacity to fight infections, is reduced in case of protein deficiencies.
- Hormones are made of proteins. Severe protein deficiency may lead to hormonal imbalances.

4. Red coloured fruits or red coloured juices help to increase Haemoglobin.

In CKD, the erythropoietin formation by the kidneys gradually reduces.

Fact:

Haemoglobin can only be increased with the help of iron and erythropoietin supplementation.

5. **All vegetables need to be thoroughly boiled before cooking.**

Fact:

Inculcate the process of "Leaching" of vegetables.

It removes the water-soluble potassium, the harmful sprays and chemicals which are used to prevent the vegetables from going bad. The process is as:

- **Wash the vegetables.**
- **Peel, scrape and chop the vegetables into small pieces, less than 1x1 inch.**
- **Soak the cut vegetable in luke-warm water for at least 30 minutes.**
- **Drain, wash again for 2–3 times, then cook.**

Refer Chapter 9 – All about Potassium.

Please follow:

- Measure water intake daily. Drink cool water. Adjust meal timings and medication timings so that the water intake is kept to a minimum and not repeated.
- Measure daily salt intake. Lesser the salt intake, lesser is the thirst and lesser the water intake. (Exceptions in this rule are the ones with low blood pressures).

- Your index finger, middle finger and thumb make a pinch on one gram of salt.
- Use the free flow, refined, iodised, sodium chloride salt. Other salts or salt substitutes may prove dangerous in case of already failing kidneys.
- Dietary protein intake must be calculated and consumed. Do not restrict or avoid proteins. Do not use protein shakes or synthetic, ready to drink proteins. They may harm your kidneys.
- Avoid fruit juices, vegetable juices or decoctions of any plants.
- Avoid coconut water, strong brewed tea or coffee, cold drinks and *sherbets*.
- Avoid dried fruits and dried nuts and oil seeds.
- Avoid items with excess salts and preservatives or chemicals as *pickles, papads, chutneys*, jams, jellies, gelatin, sauces, ketchups, ice-creams etc.
- Read nutrition--food labels on ready to eat items before buying them.

Facts to Remember

- ✓ **For CKD patients, the 24-hour urine output plus 500 millilitres of plain water intake is sufficient to remove toxic wastes from our system.**
- ✓ **Proteins in Indian diet are already on the lower limits of normal. Kindly follow dietary guidelines, do not restrict proteins.**

- ✓ Salt intake should not exceed 8 gm per day.
- ✓ Haemoglobin can only be increased with the help of iron and erythropoietin supplementation.
- ✓ Please inculcate the process of leaching.

Chapter 18

Diet in Hemodialysis Patients

Patients who are on hemodialysis usually encounter a number of challenges. They are

- Physical,
- Financial,
- Social,
- Psychological and
- Nutritional.

The key to a better quality of life on dialysis is

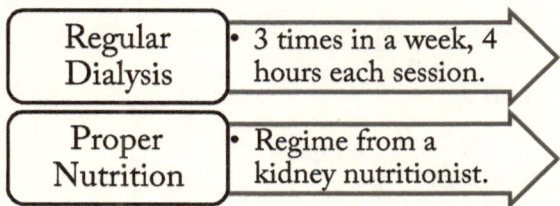

- Regular dialysis therapy and
- Good nutrition regime.

Achieving a good nutrition regime can be challenging as there are multiple aspects that need to be addressed.

This chapter is aimed at addressing various aspects of nutrition for hemodialysis patients.

When a patient is initiated on hemodialysis, he is usually confronted by a number of questions especially on diet.

The major worry or say misconception in the minds of most dialysis patients is that they need to adhere to extremely strict diets which would almost leave them starving and at the same time force them to eat things completely different from rest of family members.

However, this is not the truth.

Patients on hemodialysis can enjoy several food items and their eating pattern need not digress completely from their family members.

To achieve a better understanding of dialysis diet, let us begin with discussion on nutrients which hold nutritional implications in hemodialysis patients:

1. Fluid
2. Salt
3. Potassium
4. Protein
5. Phosphorus
6. Calories

- **What is the role of fluid in hemodialysis patients?**

As the functioning capacity of kidney goes down, their ability to handle fluid decreases resulting into its accumulation in the body.

This accumulation of fluid can lead to consequences like raised blood pressure, swelling over feet or face, breathlessness, etc.

Restriction of fluid is essential in order to avoid these complications.

The term 'fluid' includes everything that is liquid at room temperature; for example; ice.

Broadly we can classify fluids as GOOD and BAD for easy understanding.

GOOD fluids	BAD fluids
Milk	Coconut water
Beverages like tea, *ukala*, milk with *haldi* (turmeric)	Fruit juices
Varan/ dal	Cold drinks
Kadi	Slushes
Buttermilk	Soups
Soyamilk	Alcoholic beverages

- **What is it that makes some fluids GOOD while others BAD?**

GOOD fluids: These are the ones which contribute to proteins (either first class or second class).

Also, they do not contribute to build up of harmful substances in the body like potassium.

Hence, these can be taken in moderation, for example, instead of plain water, one may choose to have plain buttermilk or *ukala*.

BAD fluids: These fluids do not provide any beneficial nutrients and they contribute to build up of harmful toxins like potassium in the body.

Hence, these should be completely avoided.

- **How much fluid can be taken by dialysis patients?**

When on hemodialysis, patients are usually asked to maintain their fluid intake in between 750–1000 ml per day. This also depends on the urine output. Urine output differs from one patient to another. Hence it is difficult to generalize the fluid intake. For a better understanding, one may use a simple formula based on urine output:

Fluid intake = previous days urine output (of 24 hours) + 500 ml

Hence, if a patient has an output of 500 ml per day then the fluid intake should be 500 ml + 500 ml = 1000 ml per day which is inclusive of all liquids (tea/milk/water, etc.)

- **What is the role of salt in hemodialysis patients?**

Fluid and salt go hand-in-hand. Hence, just like weak kidneys cannot flush out excessive water, similarly they cannot flush out excessive salt.

A combination can lead to excessive fluid overload and thereby complications like breathlessness, swelling, etc.

A low salt diet is extremely essential to limit weight gain in between 2 hemodialysis sessions.

Diet in Hemodialysis Patients

- **What is the exact amount of salt that should be consumed by hemodialysis patients?**

Again, salt intake is dependent on fluid allowance.

For hemodialysis patients, it is advisable to limit salt intake to 2 grams for every 500 ml fluid allowance.

(Refer to Chapter 8 – Salt and Sodium.)

Usual intake of salt in normal individuals is approximately between **6–7 grams** and may exceed depending on the type of food choices preferred.

Salt intake increases considerably with level of dependency on packed and processed foods.

- **Which salt should be preferred by hemodialysis patients?**

This is one of the most frequently asked questions by the dialysis patients.

The type of salt does affect your blood parameters and hence it is extremely essential to keep a check on the type of salt being used in daily routine.

Normal table salt contains sodium chloride; however, there are other salt substitutes available in the market aimed at replacing sodium.

To replace sodium, the mineral used is potassium.

However, high potassium being a danger in dialysis patients, these substitutes should be completely avoided.

It is advisable to prefer only normal iodized salt for all hemodialysis patients.

- **How should potassium be controlled in hemodialysis patients?**

Potassium is a mineral in human body like sodium.

Healthy kidneys maintain potassium within its normal range in our body.

Weak kidneys cannot handle potassium.

Hence, potassium may build up in the blood.

Any extremes in the level of blood potassium can lead to heart trouble including cardiac arrest (sudden stopping of heart).

Herewith enlisted are a few general guidelines for a low potassium diet:

- Avoid coconut water and fruit juices
- Avoid soups, soup mixes especially ready to eat soups
- Avoid adding coconut to gravies, sweets, etc.
- Avoid chocolates, dry fruits, nuts and oilseeds
- Avoid salt substitutes
- Prefer moderate to low potassium cereals, *dals*, pulses, vegetables and fruits.
- Prefer leaching vegetables and *dals* in case your serum potassium is high.

- **What about intake of proteins in hemodialysis patients?**

Hemodialysis is a challenging procedure in terms of maintaining muscle mass.

A high protein diet is extremely important to compensate for the loss of protein and mainly amino acids that occur during dialysis.

It is estimated that on an average, approximately 35–70% patients face the problem of malnutrition on dialysis.

Due to malnutrition, patients are highly susceptible to infections and thereby hospitalizations.

Patients on hemodialysis need to maintain an intake of **1.2–1.3 grams protein per kg body weight per day**; with 50–70% high biological value protein.

At times, adhering to such a high protein diet may not be feasible for patients especially vegetarians and hence, they can be recommended protein supplements. These protein supplements can be in the form of powders or gels or biscuits.

A careful priority needs to be given to proteins to ensure optimal nutritional status and healthy living.

A high protein diet works even better when supported with an optimal amount of calories coming from non-protein components like carbohydrates.

In the absence of that, proteins may themselves be burnt for calorie production and may not be able to meet nutritional needs adequately.

Indian Diets in Kidney Diseases

- **How can hemodialysis patients maintain optimal protein intake?**

For non-vegetarian patients:

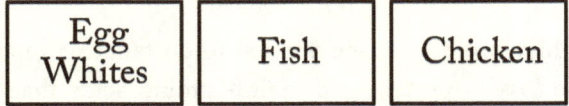

The best source of easily available and first-class protein is **egg white.**

Patients can prefer 4–6 egg whites a day including all forms, for example boiled form, scrambled form, omelet form, etc.

To maintain enough calories intake along with proteins, patients can prefer egg *parathas* or egg *biryani* or egg omelets with *chapatis*.

Another option is consuming **fish/ chicken** twice a week; approximately 3–4 small pieces (without coconut).

For vegetarian patients:

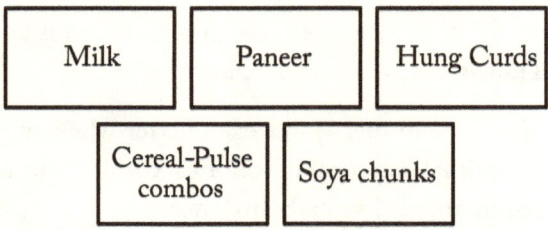

Milk and milk products make up the best source of high biological value protein; however, owing to the fluid restriction *paneer* should be preferred more than milk and curd.

Hung curd is also a good source of high biological value protein.

A better way of incorporating high biological value protein in daily diet is by using recipes which contain a **cereal and pulse combination.**

For example, *idli*-sambhar, *dosa-sambhar, khichdi*, etc.

Recipes with cereal pulse combination are higher biological value than cereals and pulses individually.

Soya chunks are an extremely useful option to incorporate protein in daily routine.

- **How to reduce phosphorus in the diet for hemodialysis patients?**

Phosphorus is also a mineral present in our body in combination with calcium.

Healthy kidneys can balance calcium and phosphorus, but weak kidneys cannot do so.

As a result, phosphorus levels start increasing.

This phosphorus usually comes from the food that we eat.

A higher level of phosphorus is harmful and can have short term as well as long term complications.

Short term complications include itching and long-term complications include weak and fragile bones, calcification (hardening) of arteries.

Hence, it is advisable to prefer a low phosphorus diet for dialysis patients.

However, the fact remains that all foods high in proteins are high in phosphorus too.

Hence, a careful selection of proteins (especially high biological value) with low levels of phosphorus is essential. One of the best forms of high biological value and low phosphate proteins is **egg whites**.

- **If maintaining a high protein and at same time low phosphorus diet is essential, then can any other remedy help?**

Yes, in such cases phosphate binders play an extremely beneficial role.

Phosphate binders are medicines that need to be eaten along with food.

These binders bind the phosphate that is released from the food and they do not allow it to be absorbed by the intestine. This phosphorus is flushed out from the body through stools. These binders need to be taken two to three times a day.

Points to Remember

- ✓ Key to good quality of life – Regular dialysis and good nutrition.
- ✓ Measure daily fluid intake. Keep it strictly according to the advice by nephrologist.
- ✓ Drink Good fluids like milk, *ukala*, soymilk, *dals*, buttermilk, *kadhi*.
- ✓ Limit salt intake. Measure salt while cooking.
- ✓ Use common salt, which is free flow, refined, iodised.
- ✓ Do not use salt substitutes.
- ✓ Keep potassium under control, by limiting the use of fruit and vegetable juices, soups, coconut water, gravies.
- ✓ Calorie intake needs to be maintained adequate to prevent protein losses.
- ✓ Protein intake should be 1.2 – 1.3 grams of protein per kilogram body weight per day.
- ✓ For vegetarians, good quality proteins can come from milk, milk products like hung curds, *paneer*, soya chunks and cereal pulse combination.
- ✓ For non-vegetarians, egg whites, deskinned chicken and steamed fish without coconut gravy is the way to go.
- ✓ Maintain fitness by daily walks, exercises and *suryanamaskaar asanas* with help of experts.

Chapter 19

Diet in Peritoneal Dialysis Patients

Peritoneal dialysis is another form of dialysis which is performed through abdomen (peritoneal cavity).

In hemodialysis, toxins are removed from the body with help of an artificial kidney (dialyzer) while in peritoneal dialysis, the peritoneal cavity of human body itself acts as a dialyzer.

Peritoneal dialysis usually is performed on daily basis hence, the body is cleared of toxins regularly.

Due to this difference in the dialysis frequency from hemodialysis (which is performed only thrice a week), diet differs from hemodialysis to peritoneal dialysis.

- **What are the key nutrients that need to be considered in peritoneal dialysis?**

In peritoneal dialysis, **protein** is one of the key nutrients that needs to be focused.

Diet in Peritoneal Dialysis Patients

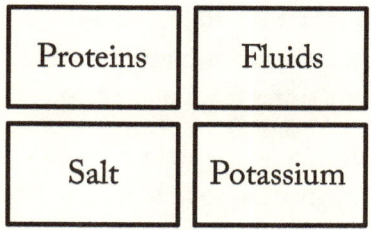

This is followed by **fluids, salt and potassium.**

Diet in peritoneal dialysis patients is comparatively liberal, to the extent that patients need to consume additional calories as well as proteins as compared to hemodialysis diet.

- **What should be the protein intake in peritoneal dialysis patients?**

In peritoneal dialysis, losses of proteins are more as compared to hemodialysis.

Five to 10 grams of proteins are lost every day on peritoneal dialysis.

Hence the intake of proteins is also advised to be higher as compared to hemodialysis.

Patients on peritoneal dialysis need to maintain an intake of **1.3–1.5 grams protein per kg body weight per day;** with 50–70% high biological value protein.

This is approximately 20% extra protein as compared to hemodialysis patients and 40–50% extra as compared to normal individuals.

Since it is not easy to be able to consume such a high protein diet, there are high chances that patients on peritoneal dialysis suffer from malnutrition.

To meet these high protein demands, proteins from natural as well as artificial sources may be needed.

- **How can peritoneal dialysis patients maintain optimal protein intake?**

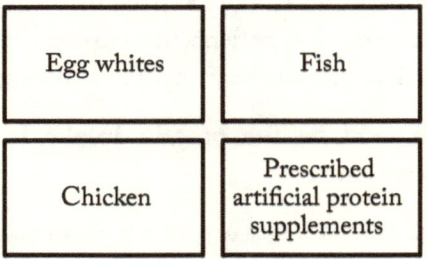

For non-vegetarian patients:

- Patients can prefer 6–8 **egg whites** a day
- **Fish**: 3–4 small pieces or **chicken**: 4–5 small pieces can be taken 2–3 times a week; (without coconut)
- **Artificial supplements** containing egg powder can be taken- 3–4 scoops a day.

For vegetarian patients:

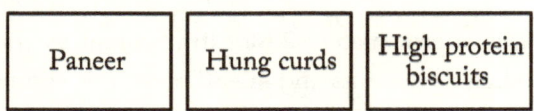

- *Paneer/chenna*: 100 grams per day
- **Hung curd**: 150–200 grams per day

Diet in Peritoneal Dialysis Patients

- Artificial supplements like high protein biscuits providing at least 10–15 grams proteins a day.

- **What about fluid and salt in peritoneal dialysis patients?**

As peritoneal dialysis is performed daily, there are less chances of fluid accumulation.

Hence, strict fluid and salt restriction is not required, unless a patient has complaints of swelling/ breathlessness/ raised blood pressure or other signs of fluid overload.

In cases with normal fluid status, the intake of fluids per day can be maintained up 2–3 liters and intake of salt up to 4 grams per day.

However, in cases with signs of fluid overload; fluid and salt intake both need to be restricted depending on the amount of fluid overload.

- **What is the role of potassium in peritoneal dialysis patients?**

Generally, as peritoneal dialysis is performed on daily basis, potassium is flushed out from the blood regularly.

Hence, restriction of dietary potassium is not emphasized unless level of potassium rises in the blood.

- **What diet instructions need to be followed if one is on CAPD and has diabetes?**

If one has diabetes, it is essential to keep a track on blood sugar values.

The dialysis exchange fluids have a lot of dextrose (sugar) which is easily absorbed in the blood and can lead to raised blood sugars.

If the blood sugar is uncontrolled, it is extremely essential to avoid simple sugars like table sugar and sugar containing food items.

If the blood sugar is controlled, it is better to avoid a simple sugar rich diet.

- **What dietary instructions need to be followed when one has to dine out?**

Need To be avoided	Can be taken
Instant soups/ soups made up of premixes	Fresh soups (limited amount-100–150 ml)
Instant gravies /gravies made up of premixes	*Idli, Dosa, Uttapam, Appam*
Alcoholic beverages	Egg omelettes, tomato omelettes, boiled egg, egg sandwiches, *paneer* sandwiches
Mocktails	Egg/*paneer*/fish/chicken based starters (boiled or barbequed)
Cold drinks	Egg/*paneer* based vegetables like *paneer bhurji*/ egg *bhurji*
Chutneys, sauces, jams and jellies	*Parathas/ Naan/ Roti/* bread

Packaged foods like instant noodles/ instant *bhels*, etc	Egg/ *paneer*/ chicken *biryani/ pulav*
Foods with excessive sauces/ gravies (extra marinated non-veg pieces)	Plain soda/ plain buttermilk/ plain *lassi* (in place of water)
	Desserts like milk cake, vanilla ice cream, *rasogulla, shahi tukda, rabdi,* etc

Chapter 20

Diabetes and Diet

India is the Diabetes Capital of the world.

Diabetes develops at a younger age in Indians. Obesity is increasing day by day. Obesity causes resistance to the action of Insulin, the hormone which controls blood sugars. Chronic diseases like hypertension, cancers, cardiovascular diseases and kidney diseases are on the rise.

Diabetic Nephropathy, meaning kidney failure due to long standing diabetes is the leading cause of Chronic Kidney Disease. Diabetic nephropathy develops in approximately 40% or more of patients with long standing diabetes. These patients have higher chances of mortality (death) due to cardiovascular problems.

Diet modification and regular exercise in diabetes is the best means to prevent our kidneys from failing. Weight-loss in obese patients prevents further damage to the kidneys by preventing protein loss through urine. Dietary modifications help prevent and/ or delay the overall complications due to

Diabetes and Diet

diabetes such as in the eyes, nerves, brain, liver, kidneys, blood vessels and the heart.

Before starting exercise and diet, a thorough nutrition assessment is performed. This includes:

- Cultural and ethnic habits
- Educational level
- Psychosocial assessment
- Socio-Economic status.
- Weight history
- Health beliefs, lifestyle
- Eating habits
- Physical activity history
- Medical history
- Laboratory reports
- Calculation of BMI
- Body fat distribution (waist measurement)
- A detailed diet history or food records are necessary for assessing eating patterns and food preferences.
- The patient's blood sugar monitoring – method, frequency and record keeping.

Let us discuss the role of Exercise and Diet in case of diabetes.

Exercise: Exercise is an important aspect of diabetes management. It helps in the following ways:

- Improves sugar control (glycaemic control) by increasing insulin sensitivity.

- Maintains body weight, reduces body fat. Fat decreases insulin sensitivity. So, reduction of fat leads to increase in insulin sensitivity.
- Reducing cardiovascular risk factors.
- Induces a sense of well-being.

Remember to take proper advice from your doctor, nutritionist and certified fitness trainer before starting any exercise program.

Diet: The purpose of medical nutrition therapy should aim to improve glycemic control without causing malnutrition.

- To control blood sugar levels
- To control blood lipid levels
- To prevent malnutrition
- To improve quality of life
- To help patients make the right food choices, by giving them the adequate knowledge about energy, nutrients and carbohydrate choices.
- To teach patients how to prevent and / or manage either low or high blood sugars and their symptoms. Prevent complications associated with these sugar changes.
- To help prevent wounds, assist in wound healing and prevent infections.
- To help prevent or delay the long-term complications of diabetes such as on the eyes, kidneys, nerves, brain and heart.

The diabetic diet therapy consists of: Three key words:

Selection, Moderation and Restriction

- Judicious **Selection** of carbohydrates.
- **Moderation** in protein intake.
- **Restriction** of total fat intake.
- Maintaining proper nutrition.
- Monitoring of total number of calories ingested.
- Obese and overweight individuals must be encouraged to reduce weight, shed off those extra fat cells, which cause insulin to become insensitive to the rising blood sugars.

General guidelines for diet in Diabetes Mellitus:

(Reference: Association of Physicians of India - API textbook of Medicine, 7th edition)

- **Calories**
  - 25 – 30 calories per kg of Lean Body Weight.
  - Reduce calories in obese and increase in underweight.

- **Protein**
  - 0.8 g per kg body weight per day.

- **Fats**
  - 20 – 25% of total calories.
  - Cooking Oil: 0.5 kg per person per month.
  - Cholesterol per day: 300 mg per day.
  - MUFA: 6 – 7% of total calories.
  - PUFA: 6 – 7% of total calories
  - Saturated fats: 6 -7% of total calories

- **Carbohydrates**
  - 55 – 60% of total calories
  - Complex carbohydrates like whole grains, pulses, beans, vegetables and salads.
  - Avoid simple carbohydrates like white sugar, bakery products which have trans fats and deep-fried items.
  - Priority should be given to total amount of carbohydrates consumed at each meal or snack.
  - Low glycaemic index foods – foods that do not lead to a sudden increase of blood sugars and are rich in fibre content- should be consumed.
  - Lis of low glycaemic index foods are whole grain cereals which are not processed or polished, vegetables, fresh whole fruits, beans and pulses, legumes and raw vegetables

- **Fruits**
  - Fresh, whole fruits.
    - ✓ Remember, kidney failure patients will have to be choosy about the fruits.
  - Strictly, no juices.

- **Dietary fibre**
  - Preferably from natural resources.
  - Indian diet is rich in fibre and generally does not require addition of fibre supplements.

- **Common salt**
  - Up to 6 – 8 gm per day.
  - Reduce intake to 4 gm per day in case of hypertension, CKD and heart problems.

- **Condiments and Spices**
    - Provide antioxidants, trace elements and minerals.
    - Some of them provide omega 3 fatty acids.

- **Nutritive Sweeteners**
    - Healthful, but must be consumed in moderation.
    - Sucrose, as in white sugars.
    - Fructose sweetened foods, fruit flavoured, can be consumed in moderation.
    - Other nutritive sweeteners: honey, maltose, dextrose, corn syrup.

- **Artificial Sweeteners: Non-nutritive**
    - Use saccharin, aspartame, sucralose, acesulfame K in limited quantity, as discussed with your physician and nutritionist.
    - Avoid artificial sweeteners in pregnancy and lactation.
    - Aspartame is contraindicated for patients with phenylketonuria.

- **Habits**
    - Avoid tobacco in any form- smoking, chewing or otherwise.
    - Avoid alcohol if possible and / or drastically restrict. It is utilised as fats and provide calories as 1 gm = 7 calories.
    - Avoid over the counter medications, especially analgesics and pain killers. These medications damage the kidneys like true enemies.

Carbohydrate Counting

- Carbohydrate counting is a meal planning approach for people with diabetes.
- The people may be on diet control or oral medications or on insulin.
- Carbohydrate is the main factor which affects the post meal blood sugars.
- More precise matching of foods and insulin is done.
- Protein and fat calories are also taken into consideration.
- There are levels of carbohydrate counting.
- We shall discuss just the basic level here.
- In this level, the person with diabetes and the nutritionist first determine the total amount of carbohydrates that will be consumed per meal or snack.
- These shall be the carbohydrate choices from starches, fruits, milk and milk products.
- You need to make choices from the list of above carbohydrates in every meal, controlling the portion sizes.
- For example, if at lunch, you wish to eat one wheat roti and one small jowar roti, instead of the routine 2 wheat rotis, then the wheat + jowar rotis (30 gm of dry flour each) are your carbohydrate choices in that meal.
  - ➤ If instead, you decide to have a mix vegetable *pulav* instead of *rotis*, then you should have *pulav* of 60 gm raw rice.

- If you wish to eat one wheat *roti* and some rice, then you should not eat the second roti, if your carbohydrate allowance for that meal is 2 carbohydrates only.
- This includes the starchy vegetables, fruits and milk choices, which are rich in carbohydrates.
- Indian meals have the *"Dal"* and "Sprouts or Legumes" component in everyday major meals, lunches and / or dinners. This is the second-class protein variety according to nutrient contents. But they have quite comparable carbohydrates in them too. These may be slightly lesser than the routine labelled carbohydrate sources. These dals and sprouts or usual sources add to the carbohydrates in Indian diets.
- In Indian diet carbohydrate counting, the dal, sprouts and *chana* or *rajma* components are to be accounted for.
- Thus, diabetic diets in Indian way should be inclusive of *dals* and sprouts for proteins, but also counted as additional carbohydrate sources.
- The problem of high triglycerides in Indians is due to the bulk of carbohydrates and second-class proteins which we have together as *Dal-Roti* or *Rajma*-Rice combinations. This may lead to consistent high triglycerides even in non-diabetics.

Moderation is the Key Here

Always remember the key – **Selection, Moderation and Restriction.**

Hypoglycemia

When blood sugar levels fall below 70 mg/dl and/or symptoms experienced are as

- Hunger
- Nervousness
- Anxiety
- Weakness
- Shakiness
- Sweating
- Light headedness
- Confusion
- Dizziness
- Falls

Severe hypoglycemia can lead to loss of consciousness.

What a person with diabetes needs to do:

- Always carry **sugar**, ORS, crystal sugars, candies, jaggery or sweets which have simple sugars in it.
- Always have some **salt** in the pocket or purse.
- Always carry a bottle of water.
- Carry an identity card with your name, address, blood group and a mention in bold letters as "I have Diabetes" in your pocket / purse/ wallet/ card holder/ on yourself always.

Diabetes Care

- **Eye care**: Keep clean. Do not use common goggles. Wash face with clean, running water.

- **Skin care:** Keep your skin moist and supple. Avoid chemicals which causes dryness and itching.
- **Foot care:** Keep your feet clean. Always wear closed footwear. Prevent injuries to feet.
- **Nail care:** Trim nails well in time to prevent infections and ingrowth of nails.
- **Personal hygiene**: Wear clean and dry clothes. Do not wear damp clothes, iron them dry, especially in monsoons.
- **Hand wash:** Doctors worldwide believe that proper handwash using soap and water prevents more than 50% of diseases due to bacteria and/or viruses. Please learn and follow proper hand washing technique.
- **Outside eating:** Choose the eat-outs judiciously. We do not wish to have food-borne infections.

Prevention of obesity by weight control and exercise is a major step towards prevention of diabetes and hence, prevention of diabetic nephropathy and other complications due to diabetes.

- Adopt and adapt to a healthy lifestyle.
- Join yoga, aerobics, weight training, dance, Zumba under certified trainers.
- Cut down on outside eating or ordering outside foods. Use your kitchen, cook with family, enjoy meals together. You will be happy as well as eating appropriate.
- Cut down on gadget time. Spend time on nature and with family.

- Cut down on lifts, enjoy climbing. Enjoy walking for short distances; you save petrol, save environment from pollution and save yourself of those extra fat globules running in your blood vessels from causing blockages, burn them down.

Eat Indian, Think Indian, Fit Indian!

Chapter 21

Diet in Kidney Stones

Kidney stones - As the name suggests these are stones that are formed in the kidneys.

They are usually formed only when there are

- Excessive waste products and
- Too little water in the body to flush them out.

It is estimated that once an individual develops a stone, he is 50% likely to develop it again over next 5 years.

The most common causes of kidney stones are:

- Drinking very little water,
- Exercising (any form) but without drinking adequate water,
- Obesity (excessive body weight),
- Eating foods that contain excessive salt and/or sugar.

As the causes of kidney stones are related to diet, it is essential to follow a diet that can lower the risk of developing stones.

1. What kind of diet should be preferred for kidney stones?

Hydration (water intake) plays key role in prevention of kidney stones.

Along with hydration, there are several other nutrients that need to be considered while discussing diet in kidney stones.

2. What does hydration therapy include?

Hydration therapy usually includes all fluids like water and fresh fluids like:

- Milk
- Buttermilk
- Soup
- Lime water
- Coconut water
- Fruit juices, etc.

Packaged fluids like packed fruit juices or soups and other beverages especially premixes (powdered, packed, ready to eat mixtures) should be discouraged.

Packed premixes of gravies and instant food items should be avoided.

It is important to note that fluids containing excessive salt or sugar and carbonated beverages like colas, iced teas, flavored drinks, etc. should also be discouraged.

3. What are types of kidney stones?

Kidney stones are mainly of 4 types:

- Calcium oxalate stones
- Uric acid stones
- Struvite
- Cystine stones

Amongst these types, calcium oxalate stones are most prevalent followed by uric acid stones. Struvite and cysteine stones are rarely observed.

The type of stone can be identified only when once flushed out from the body, these stones are sent for chemical analysis in a laboratory.

Most diet plans are prescribed by the type to stone identified. However, if identification of type of stone is not possible, hydration along with salt and sugar reduction remains the key approach.

4. What kind of diet should be followed if you have calcium oxalate stones?

Biggest thing to remember here is, calcium is not the culprit!

On the contrary, a diet containing less amount of calcium increases the chances of developing calcium oxalate stones. This is because the oxalate, that comes from the diet, does not have enough calcium to bind with in the intestines. Hence, all the oxalate in the intestine gets absorbed in circulation and reaches the kidneys where it gets deposited along with the calcium released in the urine.

Guidelines for managing calcium oxalate stones

- **Reducing salt intake.**
  This is because extra salt compels your body to lose more calcium in urine.

- **Reduce the intake of oxalate rich foods.**
  ➢ Oxalate rich foods include:
    ✓ Vegetables like spinach, beet, celery, beans, ladies' finger, capsicum, tomato, sweet potato,
    ✓ Beverages like tea, coffee, cocoa
    ✓ Fruits like grapes, currants, figs, plums and berries including strawberries, blackberries, raspberries and gooseberries
    ✓ Nuts and chocolates.

5. What kind of diet should be followed if you have uric acid stones?

Uric acid stones are formed due to intake of high amount of red meat, organ meats, alcoholic beverages, processed meat-based recipes, etc.

Hence, it is essential to adhere to a vegetarian (including fresh fruits, vegetables, dals, pulses, whole cereals, milk and milk products) diet if you have uric acid stones.

Additionally, it is important to reduce salt and sugar intake.

6. What are the general instructions for prevention of kidney stones?

- Maintain hydration of up to 3–4 liters or as prescribed by your doctor.
- Prefer hydration with **FRESH FLUIDS** only. Say no to packed fluids!
- Avoid excessive salt intake.
- Maintain a healthy weight.
- Prefer regular exercise but maintain good level of hydration while exercising (500–1000 ml per session)
- Avoid any vitamin supplementation without prescription of your doctor.

Note: The above discussion is about diet in stone disease without kidney failure. The choice of food items become complex if one has kidney failure in addition. Please consult your doctor and your nutritionist before embarking on any diet.

Chapter 22

Diet After Kidney Transplant

A diet containing solid food is begun usually on day 2 or day 3 after kidney transplant surgery.

The initial diet completely depends on the kidney function of the transplanted kidney.

Nutritional demands of the body are different during the first 4 -6 weeks post kidney transplant.

After this initial phase, nutritional demands differ.

It is essential to plan a diet with the help of a Renal Dietician immediately post-transplant in order to make the necessary changes from dialysis diet to transplant diet.

Diet instructions for first 6 weeks post renal transplant:

- **Protein:** During this stage, body requires higher proteins (**1.2 grams per kg body weight**) as well as calories to ensure good healing.
- For aiming a high protein diet:

- ➢ Prefer **first class proteins** like egg whites, milk and milk products as they can be better utilized by the body.
- ➢ Other non-veg sources like chicken can be taken. Fish has been allergenic in some cases. Especially when the post-transplant patients are on medicines like immunosuppressants, they need to avoid substances causing allergic reactions, fish being one of them, sea foods the other.
- ➢ You will require the help of your renal dietician to exactly know in what quantity it can be taken.

- **Fluid:** Once your new kidney begins to function well post-transplantation, your urine output will be good, you will not need to restrict fluids. On the contrary, you need more fluids in order to keep your body well hydrated. Your nephrologist will discuss with you about the amount of fluid needed for you. Usually, the 24-hour intake and output are measured, and a positive balance needs to be maintained. Initially, per hour urine output is measured and the color of the urine should be palest yellow or just like water. This is to ensure that the kidneys are well hydrated, flushed and working.
- **Salt:** Salt intake should be individualized as per your body demands. This will be decided by your nephrologist and then, your renal dietician can educate you how to space up that amount in your diet to make it comfortable for you.

- **Potassium:** You may not need to restrict the amount of potassium in the diet.
  - ➤ The amount of potassium to be taken depends mainly on the medications that you are on and the level of potassium in your blood. If potassium levels rise in blood, you may be asked to take a low potassium diet for 1–2 weeks.
- Strictly refrain from eating outside food and water (at least for first year after transplantation).
- Avoid eating raw food items for first 6 months; for example, salads, fruits, etc.,
  - ➤ instead prefer them in steamed form as this helps in minimizing the chances of food infection.
- Due to your medications, you may feel hungry very frequently;
  - ➤ hence, you should eat small frequent mini meals at regular intervals.
- Keep homemade mini snacks handy like roasted *chana*, roasted jowar popcorns, boiled corn, roasted *poha chiwda*, roasted *makhana*, tossed *paneer*, boiled egg whites, etc.
- Keep simple sugar like table sugar to minimum amount and avoid if you are a diabetic.

Diet instructions after first 6 weeks post-transplant till 1 year:

- After first 6 weeks, your protein level will be tapered depending on your healing.

- > After 6–8 weeks, you can have a normal protein intake – 1gram per kg body weight.
  - > If you start gaining weight at a high pace, your calorie intake needs to be adjusted as per the body weight. You need to maintain a normal Body Mass Index (BMI) post-transplant and hence if you are gaining too much weight, decreasing the calorie intake may be required.
  - > In order to avoid excessive weight gain, it is essential to perform exercise as suggested by your doctor.
- A high fiber diet helps in providing satiety (feeling of fullness) and at the same time does not contribute too much calories and helps in reducing blood sugar levels.
  - > High fiber foods like fresh fruits, vegetables, roasted whole grains, whole pulses, etc.
- Keeping weight in control also helps in prevention from future possibilities of proteinuria (protein leakage in urine), diabetes or high blood pressure.

Diet instructions after 1 year of Kidney transplant:

- After completion of first year, diet is usually unrestricted, but one needs to be careful about the nutritional side effects of certain transplant medicines which include weight gain, high blood sugar, high cholesterol.
- Depending on the side effect, you will be asked to follow dietary restrictions accordingly.

- In case you have completely healthy profile, then you need to take care of only two things:
  - ➤ Hygienic food and water
  - ➤ Regular exercise

Chapter 23

Diet in Nephrotic Syndrome – The Protein Losing Kidney Problem

Nephrotic syndrome is a condition where-in the filtering chambers of kidneys (known as nephrons) are damaged which leads to leakage of proteins in the urine.

Under normal circumstances, kidneys do not leak out urine; however, when these small filters present in our kidneys get damaged (due to several reasons), protein leakage may start occurring.

It may give rise to swelling - often noticed on legs, face or around eyes.

Along with protein leakage, patients may also have raised blood pressure and high cholesterol and triglyceride levels.

Hence, diet for nephrotic syndrome is mainly aimed at:

- Reducing swelling
- Achieving normal targets of blood lipids like cholesterol
- Achieving normal blood pressure target in patients with high blood pressure.

Dietary Instructions for Nephrotic Syndrome

A **vegetarian diet** containing fresh vegetables, fruits, cereals, milk and milk products, soya can prove to be beneficial. Herewith enlisted is a complete specification of all nutrients related to Nephrotic syndrome:

- **Fluid and salt:** In nephrotic syndrome, it is important to reduce fluid and salt intake. A **"NO ADDED SALT"** proves to be beneficial for reduction of edema as well as in achieving a better blood pressure control. Salt substitutes should be completely avoided.
- **Proteins:** Patients with nephrotic syndrome need a moderate protein diet (0.7–1.0g/ kg body weight plus the amount of proteins lost in urine) with 50% proteins from high biological value. However, it is not recommended to further reduce or increase the protein intake. In order to achieve this target, it is advisable to limit the total proteins to any of the 2–3 items from the list given below:
  - **Milk:** 150–250 ml per day
  - **Curd:** 50 grams or paneer: 4–5 small pieces per day
  - *Dal*: 1 -1 ½ medium bowl or pulses: 1 small bowl per day

- ➤ **Fish/ chicken**: 2–3 small pieces (once a week, without coconut and in roasted/ steamed/ grilled form – to reduce oil content)
- ➤ **Soya**: 20–30 grams per day

- **Potassium:** A low potassium diet is needed only in case potassium level in your blood rises. It may rise or even fall due to the side effect of some medications hence; regular monitoring of serum potassium is essential.
  - ➤ If the potassium levels are found to be low, potassium intake could be liberal in nephrotic syndrome patients.

- **Fats:** A restricted fat diet (comprising < 30% total calories, low saturated fats and high monounsaturated and polyunsaturated fats) is advisable. A plant based vegetarian diet including soy protein is found to be useful for patients to lower their cholesterol.

Chapter 24

Use of Ketoanalogues in Chronic Kidney Disease

As discussed earlier in this book, the main role of diet in chronic kidney disease (CKD) is

- to slow the progression of disease and
- delay the onset of renal replacement therapy (i.e. transplant or dialysis).
- Efforts are taken worldwide to achieve this task and one such effort is the use of Ketoanalogue.

What are ketoanalogues?

Ketoanalogues are tablets which may be prescribed by your Nephrologist.

These tablets contain essential amino acids (smallest units of proteins) but minus their nitrogen content; hence they are believed to play an important role in CKD.

In short, these tablets include all good qualities and exclude all the bad qualities of proteins; from the point of view of kidney disease.

The good qualities mainly include helping in maintaining nutrition status. The bad effects of nitrogen include becoming a part of the urea molecule. So if the amino acids do not contain nitrogen, less urea will be generated.

Hence, when these tablets are consumed, they do not lead to accumulation of nitrogenous waste products.

What is the role of ketoanalogues in CKD diet?

Ketoanalogues help by reducing the buildup of nitrogenous waste products.

They are thus, said to be delaying the progression of kidney disease.

In short, it may help in delaying the need for dialysis or transplant.

While in which class of patients these effects can be seen in best way remains a topic of research, but it is essential to know that these tablets work with specialized diets only.

For these ketoanalogues to work, patients need to be advised a low protein or a very low protein diet (as low as 0.4–0.6g/kg body weight).

Do you need to make any dietary changes if you are on ketoanalogues?

Yes, it is extremely essential to take help from a Registered Renal Dietitian before beginning with a low protein or very low protein diet.

This low protein diet needs to be strictly under supervision and guidance of a nephrologist and a registered renal dietitian.

No other patients, who are not on Ketoanalogue medications, may be benefitted by following a very low protein diet. It can lead to dangerous side effects like malnutrition, susceptibility to infection and poor outcomes in future. They may land into serious malnutrition and its complications.

A typical low protein or very low protein diet includes careful selection of foods which contain minimal proteins like rice, *sago (sabudana)*, roots and tubers, vegetables and fruits.

This diet allows minimal consumption of milk and milk products, dals, pulses, eggs, fish, chicken, etc.

How can one stay on ketoanalogues for a long period of time?

The main factor that can help one do well on ketonalogues for longer duration is providing sufficient calories from non-protein sources. In fact, keto analogues take care of all the protein requirement of the patient. That is the reason, proteins from the diet have to be cut off.

If enough calories cannot be provided or if the patient is unable to maintain an optimal calorie intake with this low protein intake, then this therapy may not be able to provide the desired results.

Hence, patient-motivation, peer support, regular follow up by a Nephrologist and regular dietary counseling play key roles in helping survive on Ketoanalogues for a longer duration.

What are the advantages and disadvantages of ketoanalogues in CKD?

Advantages

- May help in reduction of accumulation of nitrogenous waste products.
- May help in delaying the onset of dialysis or transplantation.

Disadvantages

- A low protein or very low protein diet may lead to excessive weight loss, malnutrition, increased susceptibility to infections and poor outcomes in future.
- Ketoanalogues are expensive.
- They need to be consumed in larger quantities; hence, the pill burden is high on daily basis.
- For example; an average 70 kg male may need to take 9 to 14 tablets of ketoanalogues per day, this leads to a large pill burden.

Chapter 25

Kidney Friendly Recipes

Suitable for:

- Kidney stones
- Nephrotic syndrome
- Chronic kidney disease
- Hemodialysis and Peritoneal dialysis
- Kidney transplant

Recipes for Breakfast or Snacks
Veg Rawa Chillas
Ingredients:

- Rawa(suji): 1 cup (45–50 gm)
- Finely chopped onion: ½ small cup
- Finely chopped carrot: $1/4^{th}$ small cup
- Finely chopped capsicum: $1/4^{th}$ small cup
- Finely chopped coriander: for sprinkling
- Curd: 1–2 tsp
- Ginger and green chilly paste: $1/4^{th}$ tsp
- Salt: as per daily allowance
- Pepper powder: $1/4^{th}$ tsp

Method:

- Take rawa in a deep bowl and add curd and 1 small cup water.
- Add all vegetables and masalas and mix well. Allow it to stand for 15–30 mins.
- Set the consistency by adding some more water if needed to make a thick batter.
- Now on a non-stick pan, pour the batter and set it into small round chillas (thick round shape).
- Use ½ tsp oil for each chilla and roast it from both sides till it turns golden brown.
- Serve hot with mint chutney.

Serves: 2–3 Chillas
Nutritive Value:

- Carbohydrates: 43.4 gm
- Proteins: 6.1 gm
- Fats: 10.8 gm
- Energy: 296.9 kcal
- Sodium: 21.8 mg
- Potassium: 108.1 mg
- Calcium: 51.7 mg
- Phosphorus: 184.8 mg

Jowar Rawa Upma
Ingredients:

- Jowar: 1 cup (30 - 40 gm)
- Rawa (suji): ½ cup (20 gm)
- Onion, chopped: 1 small cup
- Green peas, boiled: ½ small cup

- Carrot, chopped and boiled: ½ small cup
- Salt: as per daily allowance
- Hing: a pinch
- Curry leaves: 3–4 in no.
- Urad dal: 1 tsp
- Mustard seeds: ½ tsp
- Jeera: ½ tsp
- Oil: 2 tsp
- Lemon/curd: optional for taste

Method:

- Soak jowar overnight and boil it in a pressure cooker in the morning.
- Now in a pan, add oil, mustard seeds and jeera seeds, allow mustard seeds to crackle.
- Now add hing, urad dal and curry leaves. Mix for 1 min and then add onion. Saute it for 3–4 mins till onion becomes brown and then add boiled green peas and carrots.
- Now add cooked jowar with ½ cup water and salt.
- Mix well till upma becomes soft. Add few drops of lemon or 1 tsp curd to enhance the taste.
- Mix well and serve hot.

Serves: 2
Nutritive Value:

- Carbohydrates: 47 gm
- Proteins: 6.8 gm
- Fats: 10.7 gm
- Energy: 313.4 kcal

- Sodium: 16.1 mg
- Potassium: 121.3 mg
- Calcium: 41.2 mg
- Phosphorus: 224.5 mg

Paneer and Mixed Veg Momos:
Ingredients:

- Wheat flour(strained) or maida: 1 ½ cup
- Onion, finely chopped: 1 cup
- Cabbage, finely chopped: ½ cup
- Capsicum, finely chopped: ½ cup
- Tomato, finely chopped: ½ cup
- Paneer, grated: 2–3 tsp
- Salt: as per daily allowance
- Pasta seasoning: 1/4th tsp
- Mixed herbs and oregano: 1/4th tsp
- Red chili flakes: pinch
- Oil: 2 tsp

Method:

- Knead a soft chapatti dough using 1 tsp oil (wheat or maida dough) and keep it aside. Avoid adding salt to the dough.
- In a pan, take oil and sauté chopped onion till they turn brown.
- Add cabbage, capsicum and tomatoes and mix well. Add grated paneer.
- Now add salt, spices and seasonings. Mix well and allow this mixture to cool down.

- Now make small balls from the dough and roll it into small puris.
- Now take the filling and add it to the center of the puris.
- Dampen the edges by applying little water on the periphery and then bring the edges together and seal them by twirling them.
- Make shape of momos.
- Steam these momos in an idli cooker.
- Serve hot.

Serves: 4 Momos
Nutritive Value:

- Carbohydrates: 57 gm
- Proteins: 15.3 gm
- Fats: 17.3 gm
- Energy: 450 kcal
- Sodium: 19.2 mg
- Potassium: 321.5 mg
- Calcium: 141.7 mg
- Phosphorus: 339.6 mg

Recipes for Lunch or Dinner
Laccha Parartha
Ingredients:

- Wheat flour/ maida: 2 cups
- Wheat flour: 2 tsp (for dusting)
- Oil: 2–3 tsp
- Jeera seeds: 2 tsp
- Red chilly flakes: 2 tsp

Kidney Friendly Recipes

- Amchur powder: 2 tsp
- Oregano: 2 tsp
- Fennel seeds(saunf): 2 tsp

Method:

- Knead a soft dough from wheat flour or maida using oil (dough should be similar to a paratha dough).
- Take jeera seeds, fennel (saunf) and dry roast them on a low flame till they give an aroma.
- Now allow it to cool down and then add red chilly flakes and amchur powder.
- Now make small equal balls from the dough and roll each paratha.
- On it lightly apply oil, and then sprinkle the powder just prepared. Sprinkle it evenly all over the paratha.
- Now start rolling one end of paratha inwards making it into a pipe.
- Once done twirl one end of paratha inwards making a flower shape and seal the outer end to the paratha tightly.
- Now using wheat flour for dusting, roll this paratha again to give laccha paratha feeling. Do not roll it too thin.
- Roast this paratha on a non-stick pan using little oil.
- Serve hot.

Serves: 2–3 Parathas
Nutritive Value:

- Carbohydrates: 48.5 gm
- Proteins: 8.4 gm

- Fats: 21.1 gm
- Energy: 419 kcal
- Sodium: 14 mg
- Potassium: 221 mg
- Calcium: 33.6 mg
- Phosphorus: 248 mg

Parwal Paneer Kheema
Ingredients:

- Parwal, chopped into half: 100 gm
- Paneer, grated: 1 cup
- Onion, finely chopped: 1 cup
- Tomato, finely chopped: ½ cup
- Salt: as per daily allowance
- Oil: 2 tsp
- Jeera seeds: 1 tsp
- Turmeric: ½ tsp
- Red chilly powder: ½ tsp
- Garam masala powder: 3/4th tsp

Method:

- Take oil in a pan, add jeera and allow it to turn brown.
- Now add onion and saute it till it turns brown.
- Then add tomato and grated paneer.
- Now add salt and all masalas, mix well and then add parwal.
- Cover the pan with a lid till parwal is cooked (till it softens)
- Serve hot with phulkas

Serves: 2
Nutritive Value:

- Carbohydrates: 8.8 gm
- Proteins: 8.3 gm
- Fats: 16.5 gm
- Energy: 239.5 kcal
- Sodium: 7.8 mg
- Potassium: 183.5 mg
- Calcium: 136.4 mg
- Phosphorus: 114.1 mg

Barley and Soya Khichdi
Ingredients:

- Barley (jau): 1 cup
- Soya chunks: 4–5
- Onion, chopped: ½ small cup
- Carrot, chopped: 1/4th small cup
- Capsicum, chopped: 1/4th small cup
- Cauliflower, chopped: 1/4th small cup
- Oil: 2 tsp
- Salt: as per daily allowance
- Jeera seeds: 1 tsp
- Turmeric: ½ tsp
- Ginger and garlic paste: ½ tsp

Method:

- Soak soya chunks in hot water for 1 minute and then in cold water for 5 mins.
- Wash and drain barley. Boil it in a pressure cooker on a low flame for 2 whistles with enough water.

- In a pan, add oil, jeera and ginger garlic paste, sauté it for 1 min.
- Now add all vegetables and cover the pan with a lid. Allow all vegetables to soften.
- Now squeeze water out from soya chunks and add soya to vegetables mixture.
- Now add cooked and drained barley, salt and turmeric.
- Mix well and allow this mixture to get cooked by covering with a lid.
- Serve hot.

Serves: 2
Nutritive Value:

- Carbohydrates: 47.1 gm
- Proteins: 10.9 gm
- Fats: 12.6 gm
- Energy: 332.9 kcal
- Sodium: 16 mg
- Potassium: 74.3 mg
- Calcium: 71.6 mg
- Phosphorus: 310 mg

Salads and Accompaniments
Garlic Raita
Ingredients:

- Curd: 100 grams
- Oil: 1 tsp
- Garlic cloves: 2–3
- Jeera seeds: ½ tsp

- Red chilly powder: pinch
- Amchur powder: optional (replacement of salt)

Method:

- Beat curd thoroughly.
- Crush garlic cloves along with jeera powder and red chilly powder.
- Take oil in a small pan, add jeera and allow it to turn dark.
- Remove from flame and then add crushed garlic and red chilly powder. Mix well.
- Add this mixture to curd.
- Can add amchur powder (if needed) which can act as a replacer of salt.

Serves: 1
Nutritive Value:

- Carbohydrates: 3 gm
- Proteins: 3.1 gm
- Fats: 9 gm
- Energy: 105 kcal
- Sodium: 32 mg
- Potassium: 130 mg
- Calcium: 149 mg
- Phosphorus: 93 mg

Khaman Kakdi
Ingredients:

- Cucumber: 100–125 grams
- Dalia (split roasted chana dal): 3 tsp

- Coriander, chopped: few
- Jeera powder, roasted: 1 tsp
- Ginger green chilly paste: 1 small tsp
- Amchur powder: optional

Method:

- Chop cucumber into small pieces and set aside for 10 mins and then drain its water.
- Grind dalia coarsely and add it to chopped cucumber.
- Now add amchur powder, jeera powder, ginger green chilly paste and chopped coriander leaves.
- Mix well and serve.

Serves: 1
Nutritive Value:

- Carbohydrates: 11.2 gm
- Proteins: 3.7 gm
- Fats: 0.8 gm
- Energy: 68.3 kcal
- Sodium: 17.5 mg
- Potassium: 122 mg
- Calcium: 18.7 mg
- Phosphorus: 76 mg

Kidney Friendly Salad
Ingredients:

- Lettuce, chopped: 25 gm
- Beetroot, boiled and chopped: 10–15 gm
- Cucumber, chopped: 15–20 gm
- Green peas, boiled: 15 gm

- Carrot, boiled or capsicum or onion, chopped: 20 gm
- Paneer, small cubes: 8–10
- Corn, boiled: 2–3 tsp
- Vinegar: ½ tsp (as per taste)

Method:

- Take a deep bowl and add all chopped vegetables add vinegar, paneer, boiled corn.
- Mix well.
- Serve cold.

Note: Can add few olives and jalapenos to enhance the flavor.

Serves: 1
Nutritive Value:

- Carbohydrates: 5.5 gm
- Proteins: 6.9 gm
- Fats: 6.3 gm
- Energy: 109.2 kcal
- Sodium: 29.2 mg
- Potassium: 47 mg
- Calcium: 95.7 mg
- Phosphorus: 179 mg

Sweets and Desserts
Kurmura Chikki
Ingredients:

- Kurmura (murmura/ puffed rice): 2 cups
- Jaggery: 1 cup
- Ghee: 2–3 tsp

Method:

- Dry roast kurmura in a deep thick pan.
- Once done keep it aside and allow it to cool down.
- In same pan, take ghee, allow it to get heated and then add jiggery.
- Mix well till jiggery melts completely and starts boiling.
- Now remove from flame and add kurmura.
- Mix this mixture thoroughly well.
- Place it in a flat round plate or make small ladoos from this mixture.
- Chikki is ready.

Serves: 3–4 Chikkis
Nutritive Value:

- Carbohydrates: 103.6 gm
- Proteins: 7.5 gm
- Fats: 20.1 gm
- Energy: 625 kcal
- Sodium: NA
- Potassium: NA
- Calcium: 23 mg
- Phosphorus: 150 mg

Sweet Poha
Ingredients:

- Poha: 1 bowl
- Sugar/ jaggery: 3 tsp
- Elaichi powder: 1/4th tsp
- Ghee: 1 tsp

Kidney Friendly Recipes

Method:

- Wash poha and drain water. Soak them in little water till they soften completely.
- In a pan, take ghee and once it gets heated, add poha.
- Then add sugar or jaggery and elaichi powder and mix well. Saute for 2 mins.
- Serve hot.

Note: The original recipe contains nuts like almonds, they can be added after consulting your Dietitian. You may opt to add few strands of kesar in this recipe.

Serves: 1
Nutritive Value:

- Carbohydrates: 54 gm
- Proteins: 3.3 gm
- Fats: 5.6 gm
- Energy: 278 kcal
- Sodium: 5.4 mg
- Potassium: 76.2 mg
- Calcium: 10 mg
- Phosphorus: 119 mg

Rose Sandesh
Ingredients:

- **Paneer: 100 gms**
- **Sugar: ½ cup**
- **Elaichi powder: 1/4th tsp**
- **Rose petals: 5–6**

Method:

- Use freshly made paneer. Mash it for 3–4 mins with help of heel of palm.
- In a non-stick pan, take paneer, add sugar and elaichi powder. Mix well till the mixture becomes soft and leaves sides of the pan.
- Once done allow this mixture to cool down.
- Make small balls and flatten the ball from center.
- Garnish with rose petals in the center.
- Refrigerate it for 2 hours.
- Rose sandesh is ready.

Serves: 7–8 in No
Nutritive Value:

- Carbohydrates: 26.2 gm
- Proteins: 18.3 gm
- Fats: 20.8 gm
- Energy: 365 kcal
- Sodium: NA
- Potassium: NA
- Calcium: 208 mg
- Phosphorus: 138 mg

Some more recipes, just a list:

Remember Leaching of the vegetables, cereals and pulses before cooking.

Remember: Selection, Moderation and Restriction.

Kidney Friendly Recipes

Salads:

- Cucumber
- Beet
- Cabbage
- Pink radish
- Lettuce
- Capsicum
- Water chestnuts (Singhada, boiled but not salted)
- Carrots
- Green peas
- Cauliflower
- Onions

Flavors:

- Mint
- Celery
- Coriander, leaves and seeds
- Cumin seeds
- Dried mango powder (Amchoor)
- White vinegar
- Pepper (white and black)
- Ginger
- Garlic

Vegetables:

- Cabbage
- Cauliflower
- Capsicum
- Cucumber
- Carrot

- Corn
- Brinjal, all types and sizes
- Mushrooms
- Green peas
- Radish
- All types of gourd vegetables

Breakfast and Snacks:

- Onion Poha (Kanda Poha)
- Mix vegetable Poha (Indore style poha)
- Green peas Poha
- Upma, made of rice flour, soji, rawa or vari
- Idli, made of rawa, vari, sago, or udad dal and rice
- Uttapam, dosa without potato veggie and chutney
- Rice noodles upma
- Rice flour tikkis
- Soya cutlets with white bread, shallow fry.
- Rice porridge or rice kheer.
- Pongal, sweet or salty
- Sago and Vari chillas
- Moong dal chillas
- Rice dhoklas, khaman dhoklas
- Vegetable sandwiches
- Poha chivda
- Dahi poha
- Dadpe pohe (konkan style)
- Omelette – Egg or besan
- Ghavane (Malvani)
- Cabbage crisps
- Stuffed capsicum, not with potatoes

- Soya salad
- Soya chillas
- Thalipeeth (Rice flour, besan, singhada flour)
- Roasted masala rice papad.
- Rice flour bhakris

www.ingramcontent.com/pod-product-compliance
Lightning Source LLC
Chambersburg PA
CBHW021542200526
45163CB00014B/727